MY FIGHT, MY STRENGTH: A CHILD'S JOURNEY THROUGH CANCER

BY NYANA JACKSON

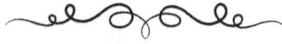

DEDICATION

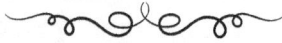

This book is dedicated to all the brave children who are facing their own battles against cancer. Your strength and resilience inspire me every day. To my family and friends, whose unwavering love and support carried me through the darkest times. To the amazing doctors, nurses, and healthcare professionals at Children's National Hospital in Washington D.C who work tirelessly to fight this disease. And to the memory of those who have fought bravely but lost the fight, you will never be forgotten.

PREFACE

I never imagined I would be writing a book like this. I was just a child, filled with dreams and aspirations, when cancer unexpectedly entered my life. It felt like a giant, dark cloud had descended, casting a shadow over my once vibrant world. But even in the darkest of moments, a flicker of hope refused to die. It was the hope of a child, the hope of a survivor, and the hope of a future filled with possibilities. This book is my testament to the strength of that hope. It is a journey through my own experience with Wilms tumor, a journey filled with challenges, triumphs, and the unwavering belief that even in the face of adversity, life can be beautiful. My hope is that this story will resonate with children facing similar battles. It is a story of courage, resilience, and the power of the human spirit. It is a story about finding strength in your support system, learning to navigate the complexities of medical treatment, and discovering the inner strength that lies within each of us. Above all, it is a story about the importance of hope, a hope that can blossom even in the darkest of times.

INTRODUCTION

It was a seemingly ordinary day, filled with the familiar sounds of laughter and the scent of freshly baked cookies. But then, the unexpected happened. A doctor's visit turned into a diagnosis that changed everything – cancer. It was a word I had heard only in hushed whispers, a word that suddenly felt heavy and ominous. Like many children facing this diagnosis, I felt overwhelmed by fear and confusion. What did this mean? How could this be happening to me? The questions swirled in my head, creating a maelstrom of anxiety.

But amidst the fear, a glimmer of determination sparked within me. I was going to fight this. I was going to be strong, I was going to be brave. And with the love and support of my family, friends, and the dedicated medical team, I embarked on a journey that would test my limits, redefine my strength, and teach me valuable lessons about life, resilience, and the power of hope.

DISCOVERY OF A NEW ADVENTURE

The sun was shining brightly, and it was a day just like any other. I was a happy little kid, full of energy, and ready to play. It was the kind of day where the world seemed full of possibilities. I could feel the warmth of the sun on my skin, smell the sweet scent of freshly cut grass, and hear the laughter of my friends as they ran and played. I was enjoying every moment of it. But then, things took a turn.

I had been feeling a little off for a few days, a strange sensation in my tummy. It wasn't pain, more like a dull ache, something that I hadn't quite been able to put my finger on. I told my mom about it, and she decided to take me to the doctor.

The doctor's office was a place I always felt a bit nervous about. I would sit in the waiting room, surrounded by the sounds of sniffling and coughing, and the smell of disinfectant that clung to the air. It felt like a place where things could get a little scary.

This time, though, it felt different. Maybe it was the strange sensation in my tummy, or maybe it was just a feeling I couldn't shake, but something felt off. The doctor, who was usually so cheerful, seemed a bit more serious than usual. After asking me a few questions about my tummy and my general health, he felt my tummy. I didn't like the way he did it, his touch seemed more intense and focused than usual. It made me feel uneasy.

The doctor looked at my mom with a furrowed brow and asked, "Would it be okay to do a few more tests, just to be sure?"

My mom, her face slightly pale, nodded slowly.

I could tell that something wasn't quite right, but I didn't understand what. It was like the air had thickened, and my world had shifted slightly, as if there was something just out of sight that I couldn't quite see.

The doctor then brought in this strange-looking machine, which was cold and felt like metal. It beeped and whirred, and I felt a strange tickle on my tummy as the machine scanned me. The doctor spent a long time looking at the screen, his brow furrowed as he studied the images that flashed across it.

"I need to have a closer look," the doctor said, his voice hushed. "Let's go for a ride."

And with that, he took me to a different place – a place that was much bigger and much more intimidating than his office. It had flashing lights, long hallways, and people in white coats everywhere. It wasn't a place I'd ever been before, and it filled me with a sense of apprehension.

As we drove there, my mom tried to keep things light. She talked about how this was just a "new adventure," and how they were going to see amazing things. But her voice was shaky, and I could tell that she was nervous.

I held onto my teddy bear, squeezing it tightly. I didn't want to let go, not even for a second. It was the only thing that felt familiar and safe. My teddy bear wasn't just a toy; it was my constant companion, my confidante, my comfort.

We finally arrived at this big, scary place called the hospital. It was full of people, all bustling about in a hurry. I was overwhelmed by the strange smells and sounds, and the vastness of the place was intimidating.

My mom, ever the reassuring presence, held my hand tightly as we walked through the corridors. She kept talking about how brave I was, and how everything was going to be okay. But I couldn't help but feel a strange knot in my stomach, a feeling that was hard to explain, like something was wrong, and I didn't know what it was.

"Don't worry," my mom said, squeezing my hand, "They're just going to have a closer look, and then we'll be back home in no time."

We arrived at a room with a large bed and a lot of machines. It looked like a scene from a movie I'd seen, a movie about aliens and doctors doing strange things to people. I felt a shiver run down my spine. The room was filled with people in white coats, and they all looked at me with a mixture of curiosity and concern.

One of them, a lady with kind eyes and a gentle voice, came over to me and introduced herself as a nurse. She smiled at me and asked my name, her voice soothing and calm.

"It's okay, sweetheart," she said, "We're just going to check on your tummy. It will be quick and painless, I promise."

My mom nodded in agreement, her face still worried, but her voice a little calmer now. She held my hand, her touch a constant reminder that I wasn't alone.

Then, the doctor, the one who'd felt my tummy back in his office, came in. He was wearing a white coat and stethoscope, and he looked serious. He told me that he needed to do some more tests to figure out what was happening.

"We're going to do a small procedure, and it will help us get a clearer picture," he said. "Don't worry, it's nothing to be scared of."

He explained everything in simple terms, trying to make me feel comfortable. But I couldn't help but feel a little nervous. What was he going to do? What was wrong with me? I felt a lump forming in my throat, a knot of anxiety tightening in my stomach.

My mom, realizing I was scared, tried to make me feel better. She talked about how brave I was, and how strong I was, and how everything was going to be okay.

The doctor and the nurse talked to me in soft voices, trying to make me feel comfortable. They showed me pictures of the machines and the tools they would use, and they explained what they were going to do. I tried to listen, to understand, but I was still a little scared.

I clutched my teddy bear even tighter, willing myself to be brave. I didn't want to cry, but I could feel the tears welling up in my eyes.

The nurse gave me a warm hug, and then they wheeled me away to a different room, where a lot of strange-looking things awaited me.

My world had changed in a way that I couldn't quite understand. The sun seemed a little dimmer, the laughter of my friends sounded a little less joyful, and the scent of freshly cut grass seemed a little less sweet. It was like a part of me had been replaced with a strange, unknown feeling - a feeling of worry and apprehension.

I held onto my teddy bear, whispering my fears and my anxieties into its soft, worn fabric. I hoped that somehow, someway, everything would be alright. And I hoped that I would be able to understand this new adventure, this new journey that had just begun. But for now, all I could do was try to be brave.

CANCER

Imagine a magical world where tiny superheroes live inside our bodies, bravely fighting off bad guys to keep us healthy. Sometimes, though, these villains, called "cancer cells," can become a bit too strong, and the superheroes need a little help to win the fight.

That's what happened to me. One day, I noticed a funny bump in my tummy. It wasn't hurting, but it felt different. My mother took me to the doctor, who, with their magic stethoscope, listened closely to my tummy and said, "Let's take a closer look to see what's going on."

That's how I learned about a big word: "cancer." It sounded scary, like a monster from a scary movie. The doctor explained that some cells in my kidneys had become a little confused and started growing too fast. They called it "Wilms tumor."

"Wilms tumor" might sound like a big, scary word, but imagine it like this: our bodies are like busy cities, filled with lots of tiny workers called cells. These cells have special jobs, like building houses or keeping the streets clean.

In my case, some of the cell workers in my kidneys were making extra houses, way more than they needed. These extra houses became the tumor, which was why my tummy felt funny. It was like having too many buildings in one neighborhood, making everything feel a bit crowded.

But just like a city has superheroes to keep things safe, my body has amazing superheroes called "immune cells." These little heroes are always working to keep me healthy, fighting off any bad guys like bacteria or viruses. But sometimes, like with my Wilms tumor, the bad guys are a little too strong for my superheroes to handle alone.

That's when the real heroes came in – the doctors and nurses. They were like a special team of superheroes, equipped with all sorts of amazing tools and superpowers to help my body fight the bad guys.

Imagine these tools like super-duper microscopes that can see the bad guys hiding in the cells. They also had magic machines that could zap the bad guys with powerful beams, weakening them and helping my superheroes fight them off. It was like a whole team of heroes coming together to save the city!

The doctors explained that I would need to visit the hospital for a while, just like when we go to the doctor when we have a cold. This way, they could keep a close watch on my superheroes and help them fight the bad guys.

At first, the hospital felt like a different world, with lots of unfamiliar machines and smells. But slowly, it started to feel like a place full of kindness and bravery.

I met other children who were superheroes too, fighting their own battles with their own teams of doctors and nurses. We laughed and played together, sharing stories about our adventures and helping each other stay strong.

Even though I was a little scared at first, I realized that I wasn't alone. My mother, my friends, and all the wonderful people at the hospital were there with me, supporting me every step of the way. They helped me remember that I was brave, that I could face my challenges, and that I would win this battle.

Just like a city needs its heroes to stay safe, my body needed its superheroes to stay strong. And just like the heroes in my favorite stories, I knew that with courage, determination, and the help of my team, I could overcome this challenge and be a superhero too.

MEETING THE HELPERS

The doors of the hospital swung open, revealing a world that felt both familiar and strange. Walls painted in calming hues of blue and green welcomed me, their surfaces adorned with playful murals of cartoon animals and whimsical landscapes. The air carried a mix of antiseptic scents and the faint aroma of freshly brewed coffee, a comforting reminder of the world outside.

My mother walked beside me, her hands intertwined with mine, her face etched with a mixture of apprehension and hope. My heart pounded a rhythm that mirrored the steady beat of the medical machines humming in the distance. It was a symphony of both fear and anticipation, a melody of the unknown.

As we approached the reception desk, a woman with kind eyes and a warm smile greeted us. Her voice, soft and calming, reassured me that everything would be alright. She ushered us into a small waiting room, where we sat on plush chairs, surrounded by families facing similar journeys.

Soon, a doctor entered the room. Her white coat seemed to shimmer under the fluorescent lights, and her stethoscope, a symbol of both hope and uncertainty, hung around her neck. She introduced herself as Dr. Seibel, a name that instantly resonated with a sense of trust.

"Hello," Dr. Seibel said, her voice gentle and reassuring. "I understand you're here because you haven't been feeling quite yourself."

She sat down, her eyes meeting mine, conveying a sense of understanding and empathy. She listened intently as my mother explained my symptoms. I felt a wave of comfort wash over me, the fear momentarily fading as Dr. Seibel's presence created a safe space for vulnerability.

After a thorough examination, Dr.Seibel explained that she wanted to run some tests. She spoke about "cells" and "tumors" in a way that was easy to understand. She mentioned the word "cancer," a word that, until then, had only been a whisper in the background of our lives.

My mother' face turned pale, her hands tightening around mine. I felt a knot of fear tighten in my stomach, a sense of confusion and uncertainty swirling within me. Dr. Seibel, sensing our anxieties, reassured us that she would be there every step of the way.

"We're going to be a team," she said, her voice filled with confidence. "We'll get through this together."

Her words, laced with kindness and hope, eased the tension in the room. We knew we were facing a difficult journey, but Dr. Seibel's unwavering optimism gave us a flicker of hope, a tiny spark in the darkness.

The hospital room became our temporary home. I spent countless hours in that room, its white walls slowly becoming familiar, the faint hum of the machines becoming a lullaby that lulled me into a state of both anticipation and dread. But, amidst the sterile environment, I discovered a world of kindness and compassion, a world where strangers became friends, and where hope flourished in the face of adversity.

There were nurses like Ms Katie , whose smile had the power to melt away any worry. She treated me not as a patient, but as a friend, telling me stories about her grandchildren and sharing her love for baking. Ms. Katie kindness was a balm on my soul, a reminder that even in the midst of darkness, there were still pockets of light.

Then there was Mr. Davis, the orderly who always had a joke ready, his laughter echoing through the hallways, a beacon of joy in the midst of uncertainty. He would wheel me down the long corridors, pointing out the whimsical murals that adorned the walls, transforming the sterile environment into a world of imagination. Mr. Davis's humor was a ray of sunshine, a reminder that laughter could be found even in the most challenging of times.

Each day, I encountered a new cast of characters – doctors, nurses, therapists, and volunteers, each playing a unique role in my journey. They were all connected by a common thread: compassion. They saw beyond the illness, recognizing the child within me, the dreamer, the adventurer, the one who longed to explore the world beyond the hospital walls.

They showered me with words of encouragement, their kind words a steady stream of strength that fueled my spirit. They celebrated my small victories, each milestone a reason to smile, a reminder that hope was a constant companion on this journey.

They spoke to me with honesty, answering my questions with clarity, easing my anxieties with their knowledge. They explained the complex world of medicine in a way that I could understand, making me feel like an active participant in my healing process.

They treated me with respect, recognizing my courage and resilience. They acknowledged my fear, validating my emotions without diminishing my strength. They empowered me to speak up, to ask questions, to be an active advocate for my well-being.

In their presence, I discovered that vulnerability was not weakness, but a strength. I learned that it was okay to ask for help, to lean on others, to allow myself to be supported.

In the heart of the hospital, surrounded by medical equipment and the constant hum of machines, I discovered a world of humanity. The hospital, once a place of fear, transformed into a haven of compassion, a place where kindness blossomed, and where hope took root. The helpers, the doctors, the nurses, the therapists, and the volunteers – they were the unsung heroes of my journey, their compassion the greatest gift of all.

THE FIRST TREATMENT DAY

The hospital room was filled with a strange mix of smells: antiseptic, disinfectant, and a faint, sweet scent of flowers. It was the kind of place that felt clinical and sterile, far from the familiar warmth of home. I sat on a small bed, my legs dangling over the edge, trying to make myself small, to disappear into the fabric of the chair. It wasn't that I was scared of the room itself. It was the unknown that loomed before me, the thing that made my heart pound in my chest and my hands sweat. This was my first treatment day, the day everything changed.

My mom sat beside me, her hand resting lightly on mine. She had this calming presence, a soft smile that seemed to brush away the anxieties that threatened to overwhelm me. But even her smile couldn't quite reach the knot of fear in my stomach. I had known about the word "cancer" for a while, but it had always been a distant concept, something I read about in books or saw on TV. Now, it was a word whispered in hushed tones in our living room, a word that had come to define my world.

The doctor, Dr. Williams, entered the room, his face kind and understanding. He had a gentle way about him, the kind of doctor who could make you feel at ease, even when your world was falling apart. He explained the treatment process in simple words, using colorful diagrams and drawings to illustrate the complex medical terms.

He talked about the medicine that would travel through my veins, fighting the tiny invaders that had taken up residence in my body. He talked about the needles that would be used to deliver the medicine, about the possibility of feeling some discomfort, but also about the strength that would come from fighting this battle.

It was all so much to take in. The word "cancer" repeated itself like a mantra in my mind, each repetition a punch to my gut. But amidst the fear, there was a flicker of hope, a small ember of defiance. I wasn't going to let this define me. I was going to fight.

The nurses, Jenny and Sarah, were like bright beacons in the sterile landscape of the hospital. They were patient and kind, their voices soft and reassuring. They showed me how to use the playroom, a small haven of color and toys, a stark contrast to the sterile white walls of the treatment room.

I held onto my mom's hand as the needle was inserted, my breath catching in my throat. The sting of the needle was nothing compared to the fear that gripped me, the fear of the unknown. But as the medicine flowed into my veins, I felt a sense of determination rise within me.

This was the beginning, the first step in a long and challenging journey. There were days to come, days of fatigue and nausea, days when the world seemed to shrink and the only thing that mattered was the ache in my bones. But I knew, even then, that I had the strength to face it all. I had my family, my friends, and the unwavering support of the medical team. And I had something else, something that burned brighter than any fear: I had hope.

The treatment day was over, but the journey had just begun.

The weeks that followed were a blur of hospital visits, needles, and scans. There were moments of laughter, of playing games with my mom in the hospital waiting area, of making new friends with other children undergoing treatment. But there were also moments of tears, of fear, of feeling overwhelmed by the weight of it all.

Sometimes, I felt like a tiny boat tossed around in a stormy sea, powerless to control the waves that threatened to engulf me. There were days when I wanted to scream, to lash out at the unfairness of it all. But then, I would look into my mother's eyes, see the love and hope reflected in her gaze, and I would find the strength to push forward.

There were days when I felt tired, so tired that all I wanted was to sleep. The medicine made me feel weak and drained, but I found ways to cope. My mom would read me stories, stories that transported me to other worlds, worlds where the word "cancer" didn't exist. She would play games with me, silly games that made me laugh, reminding me that life still held joy, even amidst the darkness.

One day, during a particularly tough treatment session, I felt a wave of panic wash over me. I looked at the machines and needles surrounding me, and I felt a sense of claustrophobia. I wanted to run, to escape the sterile white walls that seemed to close in around me.

But then, I remembered the story my mom had read me the night before, the story of a young girl who battled a dragon. In the story, the girl was scared, but she knew that she had the strength to overcome her fears. And as I looked around the room, I saw the dragon, not in the form of a monstrous creature, but in the form of my illness.

But just like the girl in the story, I had the strength to face my own dragon. I had the love of my family, the support of my friends, and the courage to fight. And I knew that I wasn't alone.

The hospital became a strange mix of familiarity and fear. It was a place of needles and scans, of waiting rooms and doctors' visits. But it was also a place where I met other children like me, children who were fighting their own battles. We shared stories, we laughed, we cried, and we found comfort in each other's company.

In the playroom, we built castles and fought imaginary wars. We played games that transported us to other worlds, worlds where the word "cancer" didn't exist. We learned to find joy in the small things, in the moments of laughter and connection, in the warmth of friendship.

The days were long, filled with the rhythmic hum of machines and the beeping of monitors. But within that routine, we found pockets of normalcy, moments of connection, and a sense of belonging.

We were all warriors, each fighting our own battles, but united by the common thread of our experiences. In that shared struggle, we found strength, hope, and the courage to keep going.

And as I looked back on those first treatment days, I realized that the journey had not only been about facing the physical challenges of cancer. It was also about finding the inner strength to navigate the emotional rollercoaster, the fear, the sadness, and the uncertainty.

It was about learning to cope, to find joy in the midst of pain, to embrace the support of loved ones, and to find the courage to keep fighting, one day at a time. It was a journey of discovery, a journey that taught me more about myself than I ever could have imagined. And I knew, as I stared out the hospital window, that the fight was just beginning, but I was ready.

FINDING COURAGE IN UNFAMILIAR PLACES

The hospital was a maze of unfamiliar sights and sounds. I was overwhelmed by the sterile white walls, the beeping machines, and the constant flow of people in white coats. I was surrounded by strangers, some smiling and kind, others rushed and preoccupied. I was scared. I missed my cozy room, my favorite toys, and my family's comforting presence. I missed the feeling of the soft grass beneath my feet, the warmth of the sun on my face, and the sweet scent of flowers in the garden.

My courage felt small, like a fragile butterfly trapped in a vast, empty space. I felt lost and alone, like a tiny ship adrift in a stormy sea. But I was determined to find my way back to shore.

One day, a kind-hearted nurse named Ms. Sarah came to my room. She had a gentle smile and a soothing voice. She brought me a colorful book filled with pictures of animals. She asked me to tell her about my favorite animal, and I chose a brave little lion. She pointed to the picture of the lion and said, "You are brave, just like this lion."

Her words were like a warm ray of sunshine, melting away my fear. They filled me with hope. I held onto her words like a precious treasure. I started to see the hospital in a different light. It wasn't just a place of needles and tests; it was a place where I could be brave, just like the lion in the picture.

I noticed the other children, like me, who were battling their own dragons. There was a girl named Lily, who had beautiful, bright eyes. She was scared of the loud noises, but she would always smile whenever she saw me. There was a boy named Alex, who loved to draw. He would share his colorful drawings of superheroes and spaceships with me, and his drawings helped me forget my worries for a while.

Together, we built a little world of our own, a world filled with laughter, games, and shared stories. We were explorers on an adventure, navigating the unfamiliar territory of the hospital. We shared our fears and our hopes, our laughter and our tears. We learned to find courage in each other, in the small acts of kindness, in the shared experiences of a journey we never expected to take.

We found courage in the simple things: the way Ms. Sarah would always read us stories, the way the nurses would sing us songs, the way the doctors would explain things in a way we could understand. We found courage in the kindness of strangers, in the cards and letters we received from our friends, in the love and support of our families.

I learned that courage wasn't about being fearless. It wasn't about pretending to be strong when I was scared. It was about facing my fears head-on, about finding ways to cope with the challenges, about finding joy in the small moments, and about never giving up hope.

Each day, I discovered new ways to be brave. I learned to use my imagination to turn the medical equipment into friendly robots and the hospital room into a magical castle. I learned to find humor in the silly things, like the doctor's funny hats or the nurse's silly jokes. I learned to find strength in the love and support of my family and friends.

My journey through the hospital was long and difficult, but it was also filled with moments of courage, resilience, and hope. I learned that even in the most unfamiliar places, we can find courage within ourselves and in the kindness of others. And I learned that even the most challenging journeys can lead to unexpected growth and discovery.

I learned that courage isn't just about facing fear, but about embracing life with a positive attitude. It's about finding joy in the simple things, celebrating small victories, and never giving up hope. And it's about sharing our stories, our struggles, and our triumphs, knowing that we can inspire others to find their own courage and strength.

My journey through the hospital taught me that courage is a journey, not a destination. It's a constant process of growth and learning. And I am grateful for every lesson I learned along the way.

One day, I will be back home, playing in the garden and running through the fields. But I will never forget the lessons I learned in the hospital. I will never forget the courage I found within myself and in the kindness of others. And I will always remember that even in the most unexpected places, we can find the strength to overcome anything.

THE FIRST LINE
OF SUPPORT

The first people who stand by you, holding your hand through the twists and turns of your journey, are your family. They are your anchor, your constant source of love and strength. They are the ones who understand your fears, celebrate your victories, and offer a shoulder to cry on when the world seems too much to bear.

Remember the day you were diagnosed? The world felt like it was spinning, and the doctor's words echoed in your ears. Maybe you were scared, maybe you were confused, but one thing was for sure: you weren't alone. Your parents, siblings, grandparents, aunts, uncles – they were all there, holding your hand, their eyes filled with love and concern.

They became your rock, your steady presence in a whirlwind of emotions. They went with you to every appointment, explaining things you didn't quite understand, holding your hand during difficult procedures, and whispering words of comfort when the fear threatened to engulf you.

It wasn't always easy for them either. They felt the same fear you did, the same uncertainty, the same weight of the unknown. But they masked it, they put on a brave face for you, because they knew you needed them to be strong.

They learned to navigate the medical world alongside you, decoding doctor's jargon, understanding treatment plans, and advocating for your best interests. They became experts in your condition, your medications, your needs.

They became your champions, fighting for you in ways you couldn't fight for yourself. They researched the latest advancements, explored alternative therapies, and connected with other families who understood the journey you were on.

Your family became your cheerleaders, celebrating every small victory, every milestone you achieved, every hair that grew back after chemo. They were there to offer a warm hug when you felt tired, a playful joke to lift your spirits, a comforting presence to remind you that you weren't alone.

They might have brought you your favorite books, movies, or games to help you pass the time in the hospital. They might have made you laugh with silly stories or funny faces when the world felt too serious.

They might have created a special routine, a bedtime ritual, or a family tradition just for you, to bring a sense of normalcy into your life.

And when the world felt too heavy, when the burden of treatment felt overwhelming, they were there to hold you, to listen without judgment, to simply be there for you.

They may have struggled to understand your emotions, your fears, your frustrations. They might have said the wrong thing sometimes, but they always meant well. They were learning too, learning to understand the complexities of this journey, learning to be the best support they could be for you.

And sometimes, the best support comes from the simplest things. A warm hug, a gentle touch, a quiet presence in the room. It's the unspoken language of love, the understanding that words sometimes fail to express.

Remember, your family isn't just there to care for you physically; they're there to care for you emotionally too.

They are the safe space where you can be vulnerable, where you can cry and laugh, where you can be your authentic self without fear of judgment.

So, lean on your family. Let them love you, support you, and care for you. They are your biggest allies in this battle.

Family is the foundation of your support network, the bedrock upon which you build your strength and resilience. They are the constant in a world that can feel chaotic and unpredictable. They are the ones who will always be there, no matter what.

But remember, while they are your first line of support, your family isn't the only one. There are other people who are here to help you on this journey.

The next chapter will introduce you to a whole world of support waiting to be discovered.

NEW FRIENDS IN
UNEXPECTED PLACES

The hospital waiting room wasn't exactly the place I envisioned making new friends. It was filled with the scent of disinfectant and the constant hum of machines, punctuated by the occasional muffled cry from a child. Yet, it was there, in that seemingly sterile environment, that I discovered an unexpected bond with other children who, like me, were facing their own battles.

One day, while I sat listlessly watching cartoons on the small TV in the playroom, a little girl with a bright red headband approached me. Her name was Lily, and her sparkling blue eyes held a mixture of curiosity and caution. We were both waiting for our chemo treatments, and the shared experience seemed to create an unspoken understanding between us.

Lily was a whirlwind of energy, bouncing around the room, her giggles echoing off the walls. At first, I found her a bit overwhelming. I was used to spending most of my days in bed, reading books or watching movies, my world shrinking to the confines of my hospital room. But Lily's infectious laughter and playful antics slowly drew me out of my shell.

We started playing board games, sharing stories, and drawing pictures together. We even had secret handshakes and code words, making the hospital hallways feel less like a medical institution and more like our own private playground.

Lily had been battling leukemia for almost a year, and she was a seasoned veteran of the hospital routines. She knew the best places to hide from the nurses, which toys were the most fun, and how to make the most of the limited space. I learned a lot from Lily, not just about how to navigate the hospital, but also about how to find joy in the midst of difficult times.

We were two kids on a shared journey, each with our own anxieties and fears, but with a growing sense of camaraderie. We understood each other's struggles in a way that no one else could. We found solace in each other's company, in the shared laughter and tears.

One afternoon, Lily told me about her favorite storybook, a tale about a brave knight who fought a dragon. She said that the dragon was like her cancer, a scary beast that she had to conquer. But the knight, she explained, wasn't afraid. He faced the dragon with courage and eventually defeated it.

Lily's story struck a chord within me. It reminded me that even in the face of fear, there was always a way to find strength. It gave me the courage to face my own battle, to see myself as a brave warrior fighting for my own life.

Our friendship didn't just happen within the hospital walls. We also connected with each other's siblings, forming a kind of extended family of sorts. Lily's brother, Max, was a year older than me and loved to play video games. We spent hours strategizing and competing, the joy of the game momentarily erasing the reality of our situation.

Max's younger sister, Emily, was a chatterbox, always bubbling over with stories and jokes. She was a constant source of laughter, a reminder that even amidst the pain and uncertainty, there was still room for lightheartedness.

Together, the four of us formed a little world within the hospital, a haven of friendship and shared experiences. We shared our joys and sorrows, our hopes and fears. We celebrated each other's milestones, big and small, from successful treatments to getting a new toy.

Our friendship was a lifeline, a source of strength and comfort in a time when we needed it most. It taught me that even in the most challenging situations, there was always room for connection, for love, and for friendship.

One day, Lily's treatment was deemed successful, and she was finally able to go home. I was happy for her, but I couldn't help feeling a sense of loss. We had become so close, our friendship a constant in my life.

However, even though Lily wasn't there physically, our connection remained. We wrote letters and sent each other cards, staying in touch with each other's lives. And when I saw her again, months later, it was like no time had passed at all.

Our friendship, forged in the crucible of shared adversity, taught me the power of human connection, the importance of finding joy in the face of hardship, and the unwavering strength that comes from having someone to share the journey with. It taught me that even in the most unexpected places, friendship can bloom and blossom, reminding us that we are not alone in our struggles.

THE POWER OF KIND WORDS

The school bell rang, signaling the end of another day. I walked out, my backpack heavy with books, but my heart even heavier with the news of my diagnosis. It felt like everyone else was moving on with their lives, while I was stuck in a hospital room, battling a big, scary word – cancer.

The thought of going back to school felt overwhelming. What would my friends say? Would they look at me differently? Would they understand?

My mother knew I was struggling. She tried to reassure me that my friends missed me and would be happy to see me back. But the fear still lingered.

One afternoon, while lying in my hospital bed, I received a small package. It was a letter from my best friend, Sarah. Her handwriting was neat and bubbly, just like her personality.

"Dear Nyana," she wrote, "I miss you so much. School isn't the same without you. We miss your jokes and your stories. We miss playing with you at recess. Don't worry about missing school. We'll be here when you get back."

The simple words, filled with warmth and love, melted my fears. I felt a surge of strength, a wave of hope, washing over me. Sarah's letter wasn't just a letter; it was a lifeline, a reminder that I wasn't alone.

The next day, I received another package. This time, it was from my classmate, Daniel. He had drawn a picture of a superhero, with a cape and a big smile. Below the drawing, he wrote, "This is you, Nyana. You're a superhero because you are strong and brave."

Daniel's drawing made me laugh. I wasn't a superhero, but his words touched me. It was as if he saw the warrior inside me, the spirit that wouldn't give up.

Days turned into weeks, and my inbox was flooded with messages and drawings from my friends. They sent me jokes, riddles, and stories to keep my spirits up. They even started a "Get Well Soon" campaign at school, with everyone signing their names on a giant poster.

One day, I received a video message from the entire class. They were all singing my favorite song, "You Are My Sunshine." The video was a bit shaky, but the love and warmth shining through their smiles were crystal clear.

Their words, their gestures, their presence – they were all like warm blankets wrapped around me, comforting me, reminding me that I was loved, that I was supported, that I wasn't alone in this fight.

Their messages were a beacon of hope, a testament to the power of human kindness. They showed me that even when I was physically away, I was still connected to them, to the world, to life.

Their messages weren't just words on paper; they were a force of love, a reminder that even in the darkest of times, kindness can be a powerful light, a beacon of hope, a source of strength. They helped me realize that even though I was going through a difficult journey, I wasn't fighting alone. I had a whole army of love surrounding me.

In the face of a daunting battle, these messages from my friends were more than just words; they were weapons of hope, shields of support, and reminders that I was loved, cherished, and not alone in this fight.

This experience taught me a valuable lesson: the power of kind words, the strength of human connection, and the enduring impact of love. It taught me that true friendship knows no bounds, that it can reach across miles and overcome any obstacle. It taught me that even in the darkest of times, a simple act of kindness can bring light, hope, and strength.

As I continued my treatment, those messages continued to be my source of strength. They were a constant reminder that I wasn't just battling cancer, I was battling with love, support, and a community of caring hearts.

One day, my doctor called me into his office. "You're doing great," he said, with a smile on his face. "Your strength and resilience are inspiring."

I knew that my strength came from within, but I also knew that it was fueled by the love and support of my friends, my family, and the kindness of people I hadn't even met. Their words had given me the courage to fight, the strength to persevere, and the hope to believe in a brighter future.

This journey has taught me that the power of kind words is immeasurable. They can lift spirits, inspire hope, and bring comfort in times of need.

The words of my friends were more than just words; they were acts of love, whispers of hope, and reminders that I was not alone. They were my lifeline, my strength, and my inspiration. They reminded me that even in the midst of darkness, kindness can shine through, bringing warmth, hope, and a belief in the power of love to overcome any challenge.

A COMMUNITY COMES TOGETHER

The news of a community coming together spread like wildfire. It started with a small gathering in our backyard, a potluck dinner organized by our neighbors to show their support. It was heartwarming to see familiar faces, the laughter and chatter filling the air, a comforting reminder that we weren't alone in this fight.

Then came the fundraiser – "A Night for Hope," they called it. The local school auditorium was transformed into a vibrant space, buzzing with energy. People from all walks of life – teachers, shopkeepers, families, even complete strangers – came together, their faces etched with concern and a shared desire to help. There were food stalls, games, and live music. The air was filled with the scent of popcorn and the sound of children's laughter, a stark contrast to the sterile environment of the hospital.

The highlight of the evening was the silent auction. Donated items – everything from handcrafted pottery to weekend getaways – filled the tables, each bid whispering a promise of hope and support. The auctioneer's voice reverberated through the hall, each bid a testament to the community's unwavering kindness.

Beyond the immediate support, the community's efforts extended to practical help. Volunteers from the local church delivered meals to our house, relieving my mother of the burden of cooking during those challenging times. A group of teenage girls organized a "card drive," sending me cheerful messages and colorful drawings that filled my hospital room with warmth and joy. Even the local bakery sent us a box of freshly baked cookies, a small gesture that brought a wave of comfort and sweetness.

As the days turned into weeks, the community's support became a lifeline. It wasn't just the tangible help, but the feeling of being embraced by a network of caring individuals who had never met us before. It felt like a giant, invisible hand reaching out, whispering words of encouragement and strength. Their unwavering support was a constant reminder that we weren't facing this challenge alone.

I remember one particular day, during a particularly tough treatment session, when a group of children from my school came to visit. They had created a giant card filled with colorful drawings and heartfelt messages. Each message was a tiny burst of sunshine, reminding me of the love and support surrounding me. They told me stories, played games, and made me laugh. For a few precious hours, the hospital walls seemed to fade away, and I felt a sense of normalcy, a reminder that life could still hold moments of joy and connection.

The community's efforts weren't just about providing support; it was about creating a sense of belonging, reminding me that I wasn't just a cancer patient, but a child, a friend, a member of a loving community. The community rallies, the fundraisers, the acts of kindness, all were a testament to the power of human connection, reminding me that even in the face of adversity, hope and strength can be found in the most unexpected places.

One event that stands out in my memory was a "Braveheart Day" organized by the local YMCA. The entire community, from toddlers to senior citizens, gathered at the park for a day filled with fun activities. There were bouncy castles, face painting, and a giant picnic lunch. The day culminated in a symbolic release of balloons into the sky, each balloon carrying a message of hope and courage. As I watched the colorful balloons drift into the endless blue sky, I felt a sense of liberation, a reminder that even though the journey was challenging, there was a possibility of joy and hope waiting on the other side.

The community's support wasn't just about providing tangible help; it was about offering a sense of belonging, reminding me that I was not just a cancer patient but a child, a friend, a member of a community. It was about creating a space where I could be myself, where I could share my fears and hopes, and where I could feel loved and supported.

The impact of the community's support went beyond the immediate challenges of treatment. It instilled in me a profound sense of gratitude and a belief in the inherent goodness of humanity. It showed me that even in the darkest of times, there are people who are willing to step up, offer a helping hand, and remind you that you are not alone. It was a lesson that stayed with me long after the treatment was over, a reminder that the power of community can truly make a difference.

Beyond the individual acts of kindness, the community's efforts also served to raise awareness about childhood cancer. The fundraisers, the events, the articles in the local newspaper, all helped to shed light on this often-forgotten disease. They highlighted the needs of children like me and the importance of research and funding for finding a cure.

The impact of the community's efforts extended far beyond me. It fostered a sense of unity, reminding us all that we are connected, that we share a common humanity, and that we have the power to make a difference in each other's lives. It showed me that even in the face of hardship, hope and strength can be found in the most unexpected places.

The community's support wasn't just about offering a helping hand; it was about building a network of love and support, a network that would help me navigate the challenges of my journey, and ultimately, emerge stronger on the other side. It was a testament to the power of human connection, reminding me that even in the darkest of times, there are people who are willing to step up, offer a helping hand, and remind you that you are not alone. This sense of community, this shared experience of strength and hope, became a vital part of my healing journey.

FURRY FRIENDS AND COMFORT GIVERS

In the midst of the whirlwind of treatments, hospital visits, and anxieties, a familiar presence brought a comforting warmth – the unwavering love of our furry companions. For many, pets are more than just animals; they are loyal friends, steadfast companions, and unconditional sources of love. They have an uncanny ability to sense our emotions and provide solace when words fail.

Remember the days when I was feeling overwhelmed by the hospital environment, the sterile smells, and the constant buzz of activity? My pet, a fluffy tabby cat named Whiskers, would curl up on my lap, purring softly. His gentle presence calmed my nerves, and the rhythmic rumble of his purr was like a soothing lullaby. In those moments, I found myself lost in the simple joy of his company, momentarily forgetting the anxieties that plagued my mind.

Whiskers wasn't the only furry friend who brought me comfort. I recall a time when I was feeling particularly down, battling the side effects of chemotherapy. My dog, a playful golden retriever named Sunny, came bounding into my room, his tail wagging furiously. The sight of his happy face and the infectious joy in his eyes lifted my spirits. Sunny's unwavering love and enthusiasm, his playful antics, and the simple act of his being there, filled me with a sense of hope and resilience that I desperately needed.

Pets, especially dogs, are often called "man's best friend," and for good reason. Their unconditional love and playful nature have a remarkable ability to lighten even the darkest days. When I was feeling weak and tired, Sunny would encourage me to go for walks, reminding me that even a little bit of exercise could do wonders for my mood and energy levels.

The bond between children and pets is especially profound. For a child navigating the complexities of cancer, having a loyal pet by their side can make a world of difference. The bond between a child and their pet provides a sense of security, stability, and unconditional love in an environment that can feel uncertain and overwhelming. Pets can offer a sense of normalcy and routine, reminding them of the simple joys of life, even during difficult times.

Imagine a child, perhaps struggling with the pain of needles or the anxieties of a new treatment. Their pet might cuddle up next to them, offering a comforting presence and a sense of safety. The simple act of petting their furry friend can be a source of distraction, allowing them to momentarily forget about their fears and anxieties.

The love and companionship of pets can even extend to other members of the family. They can provide a much- needed distraction for siblings who may be struggling to cope with the changes brought about by their loved one's illness.

The power of pets is not just about providing emotional comfort; it can also extend to physical well-being. Studies have shown that interacting with pets can reduce stress, lower blood pressure, and even help manage chronic pain. The simple act of petting a furry friend can release oxytocin, a hormone associated with bonding and relaxation, promoting a sense of calm and well-being.

It's important to note that not everyone has the opportunity to have a pet, and that's perfectly alright. The love and support from family and friends can be just as comforting and valuable. However, for those who do have pets, their presence can be a source of incredible strength and resilience during challenging times.

In my journey, pets played a vital role in providing love, companionship, and a sense of normalcy. They were my furry therapists, my silent companions, and my unwavering source of strength. If you are facing a difficult time, remember the joy and comfort that your furry friend can provide. Allow them to be a source of love and support, reminding you that you are not alone.

As I reflect on my journey, I recognize the profound impact that pets have had on my life and the lives of so many others. They are reminders that even in the darkest of times, love, joy, and companionship can be found in the most unexpected places. The unconditional love of a furry friend can be a beacon of light, a source of strength, and a reminder of the beauty that exists in the world, even amidst the challenges.

UNDERSTANDING THE TREATMENT PLAN

The treatment plan was like a map leading us through a maze of tests, scans, and medications. It wasn't always easy to understand, but the doctors and nurses were there to explain everything in a way I could grasp. It was like a big adventure with lots of different steps, and I had to trust them to guide me through it.

They talked about something called "chemotherapy," which sounded a bit scary, but it was actually just a special medicine that helped fight the little warriors in my body that were causing trouble. They told me it was like giving my body a superpower to defeat them. The medicine came in different forms, like pills, injections, and even a special kind of IV drip that flowed into my veins like a magical potion.

They explained that the medicine would make my body strong and able to defeat the tumor, but it would also make me feel tired and sometimes a bit sick. It was like my body was working extra hard to fight the bad guys, and it needed a break sometimes. But they promised that I would be able to bounce back with lots of rest and good food.

Some days, I felt like a superhero with incredible strength. I could play with my friends, read books, and even draw amazing pictures. But other days, I felt tired and needed to rest. I learned to listen to my body and take breaks when I needed them. It was like having a secret code that told me when it was time to recharge my superpowers.

The doctors also talked about something called "radiation therapy," which sounded a bit like a magic beam that could zap the bad guys. It wasn't scary at all, it was like a short trip in a special room with a machine that made a soft buzzing sound. It felt a bit warm, like a gentle hug from a sunbeam. They said it would help stop the tumor from growing, and it would be like giving it a little freeze.

I learned that the treatment was like a journey with its own ups and downs, but it was a journey I had to take to get back to feeling strong and healthy again. There were days when I felt happy and energetic, and there were days when I felt tired and a bit down. But I knew that every step I took was bringing me closer to being healthy again.

During the treatment, the doctors checked up on me regularly with blood tests, scans, and checkups. It was like a special mission to make sure everything was going according to plan. They would talk to me about how I was feeling and answer any questions I had. It was like having a team of superheroes working together to help me get better.

The most important thing was to stay positive and focus on getting better. My family, friends, and even my teachers helped me do that. They reminded me of all the things I was good at and all the things I could still enjoy. It was like having a cheerleading squad that never gave up on me.

I also learned to find joy in the little things. A funny joke, a good book, or even a warm hug from a loved one could make me feel better. It was like discovering a whole new world of happiness that I hadn't noticed before.

The treatment process was a long and sometimes difficult journey, but I learned so much about myself during that time. I learned about the strength I had inside, the power of hope, and the importance of support from the people I loved. It was like a secret code that unlocked a new level of courage and resilience within me.

Celebrating Small Victories

The journey of treatment wasn't just about battling the big enemy. It was also about celebrating the small wins along the way. Each time I woke up feeling a little better, or could manage to play for a few minutes longer, it felt like a victory.

Remember those fun stickers they give you at the doctor's office? Every time I went for a check-up and everything was good, I got a new sticker, and it felt like a little badge of honor.

These small wins were a reminder that I was fighting, I was getting stronger, and I was moving closer to feeling completely myself again.

Handling the Tough Days

There were days, of course, when the treatment made me feel tired, weak, and even a little bit scared. It felt like the bad guys were winning, and I felt like I was stuck in a dark, scary place.

During these times, it was really important to have people around me who understood what I was going through. My mother was there for me every step of the way, and she helped me find ways to feel better. She reminded me that I was strong, that I was brave, and that I was going to get through this.

Sometimes, even with her love and support, those tough days were still hard. That's when my imagination came in handy. I used my imagination to create my own world where I could be anything I wanted to be. I imagined myself as a powerful superhero who could defeat any enemy, or a brave explorer who could conquer any obstacle.

My favorite way to escape those tough days was by reading books. I got lost in stories about adventure, magic, and friendship. It helped me forget about my worries and focus on something positive.

The Importance of Rest and Play

Rest and play were also important parts of my treatment journey. It was like giving my body a chance to catch its breath and recharge its batteries. I learned to listen to my body and take breaks when I needed them.

My mother made sure I got plenty of sleep, even though I didn't always want to. It was like a magical potion that helped me feel stronger and more energetic the next day.

And when I felt up to it, I played with my friends, read books, and even did some art projects. It was like a way to remind myself that I was still a kid, even though I was going through something difficult.

Keeping the Spirit High Through Creativity

Art and imagination played a huge role in helping me stay positive. It was like a secret weapon that helped me face the challenges of treatment.

Drawing and painting allowed me to express my feelings and emotions in a creative way. It didn't matter if my drawings were perfect or not, the important thing was that they helped me feel better.

I also loved to write stories and poems. It was like creating my own little world where I could be anyone I wanted to be.

My imagination was my superpower, helping me through the tough times and reminding me of the joy and wonder in the world.

CELEBRATING SMALL VICTORIES

It's hard to imagine how someone can find joy in the midst of such a difficult journey. The truth is, it's not about finding happiness in a big way. Instead, it's about finding little moments of joy within the everyday routine of treatment. These small victories can make a huge difference in your overall well-being and help you stay positive.

For me, a small victory might be as simple as getting out of bed and taking a walk around the hospital floor, even if it's only for a few minutes. The fresh air and the change of scenery always helped me feel a little bit more alive. Another small victory was being able to eat a meal without feeling nauseous. Those days were like a little celebration, and I savored every bite.

Remember those tiny rubber ducks that came with every bath? Those simple toys gave me immense joy. I'd make up stories about them, their adventures in the bathtub, and how they were fighting off germs. The laughter that came with it was a little ray of sunshine on gloomy days.

Another way to celebrate small victories was through art. Drawing or painting was my way of expressing myself when words failed me. Every stroke of the brush felt like a small win. Even if the artwork wasn't perfect, it was a way for me to release some of the emotions I was carrying.

One of the most unexpected small victories was simply connecting with other kids going through similar treatments. Sometimes, it was as simple as sharing a smile or exchanging a few words. We understood each other in a way that no one else could. And those moments of shared understanding were incredibly valuable.

I also found a lot of joy in the small acts of kindness from others. Maybe it was a card from a friend, a warm hug from a family member, or even a stranger offering a kind word. Every little act of kindness felt like a small beacon of hope, reminding me that I wasn't alone in this journey.

It's important to remember that there will be tough days too. There will be times when you feel like giving up, and that's okay. It's part of the journey. But even on those tough days, try to find at least one small victory to celebrate. It might be as simple as taking a deep breath, enjoying a moment of silence, or reading a favorite book.

These small victories, though seemingly insignificant, are like tiny seeds that sprout into a beautiful garden of hope and resilience. They remind us that even in the darkest of times, there is always something to be grateful for. So, celebrate those small victories, no matter how small they seem, and let them fuel your courage and determination as you navigate this challenging journey.

HANDLING THE TOUGH DAYS

The days of treatment weren't always sunshine and rainbows. Sometimes, the fatigue would be so overwhelming that even getting out of bed felt like climbing Mount Everest. The nausea would come in waves, leaving me feeling like I was on a rollercoaster that wouldn't stop. There were times when the pain felt like a thousand tiny needles pricking my skin, and the chemo would leave me feeling weak and depleted.

It's important to remember that everyone experiences treatment differently. What worked for me might not work for someone else, and that's okay. The key is to find what helps you cope with the tough days.

One of the things that helped me most was having a good support system. My mother is my rock, always there to hold my hand and whisper words of encouragement. My siblings, even though they were younger, would come up with silly jokes and games to make me laugh. Having their love and support made a world of difference.

But it wasn't just my family. My friends at school were also amazing. They sent cards, drew pictures, and even organized a fundraiser to help my family with expenses. It was incredible to see how much they cared, even though they didn't fully understand what I was going through.

Another thing that helped me was finding ways to distract myself. Sometimes, reading a book or watching a movie would take me away from the reality of my situation. Other times, I would find myself lost in a world of my own imagination, creating stories and characters that filled my mind with joy and wonder.

The doctors and nurses at the hospital were also incredibly helpful. They would always take the time to explain things to me in a way that I could understand. They were patient with my questions and never made me feel silly for asking them. They were more than just medical professionals; they were my friends and my confidants.

But even with all of this support, there were still days when the sadness and fear would feel overwhelming. On those days, I would talk to my mother or a therapist about how I was feeling. It was okay to let my emotions out, to cry if I needed to, and to simply acknowledge that I was struggling.

The most important thing was to remember that I wasn't alone. There were countless others who had walked the same path, and they had found strength and resilience on the other side. There were support groups, online forums, and books written specifically for children going through cancer treatment.

These resources helped me feel connected to a community of people who understood what I was going through. They offered words of encouragement, shared coping strategies, and helped me realize that even though this was a tough battle, it wasn't impossible to win.

Here are some specific strategies that helped me get through the tough days:

Finding a Creative Outlet: I always loved drawing, so I would spend hours sketching fantastical creatures and landscapes. It helped me escape the confines of the hospital walls and allowed my imagination to soar. It didn't have to be drawing; maybe it's writing, playing music, or anything else that allows you to express yourself creatively.

Mindfulness Techniques: My therapist taught me how to practice mindfulness. It helped me stay grounded in the present moment, focusing on my breath and my senses. There are simple exercises you can do, like focusing on the feeling of your feet on the floor, or counting the sounds you can hear around you.

Keeping a Gratitude Journal: Every day, I would write down three things I was grateful for. It could be anything from the taste of a delicious meal to the kindness of a nurse. Focusing on the good things in my life helped me to see the world in a more positive light, even amidst the challenges.

Setting Small Goals: Instead of focusing on the overwhelming task of beating cancer, I would set small, achievable goals. It could be something as simple as getting out of bed and taking a short walk, or reading a chapter of a book.

Sometimes, the toughest days felt like they would never end. But with each sunrise, a new opportunity for strength and hope presented itself. Remember, you are stronger than you think. You have the power to get through this, and you will come out of it even more resilient and determined than before.

THE IMPORTANCE
OF REST AND PLAY

The hospital, with its sterile walls and beeping machines, wasn't exactly a playground. But even in that space, a place where fear sometimes lingered, there were pockets of joy, whispers of laughter, and the magic of imagination. It was crucial, especially during treatment, to carve out moments of playfulness, to allow ourselves to escape the reality of needles and tests for a little while.

Remember those days when you felt like a superhero, your cape flowing in the wind as you battled evil villains? Maybe you were a princess in a faraway castle, surrounded by loyal subjects, or a brave explorer trekking through uncharted jungles. We all have those stories inside us, and they can be powerful tools for coping with challenges.

The doctors and nurses, those valiant warriors in their white coats, understood this too. They were the ones who brought in the crayons and coloring books, the puzzle sets, and the board games. They knew that laughter and play could help mend a broken spirit, just like a good bandage could heal a wound. They encouraged us to draw, to sing, to dance, to let our inner child come out and play.

Sometimes, even the smallest act of play could feel like a big adventure. Remember how we used to pretend our hospital beds were pirate ships, sailing across the vast ocean of the hospital floor? We'd gather our stuffed animals as our loyal crew, and with a few well-placed pillows, we'd build our own pirate ship fortresses, battling imaginary sea monsters and searching for hidden treasures.

Even when we weren't feeling our best, the nurses would make sure we had toys to keep us company, and the doctors would tell us stories about brave knights and courageous princesses who fought their battles with bravery and grace. Those stories, woven into our imagination, gave us strength to face our own challenges.

But play wasn't just about games and toys. It was also about finding joy in simple things, like watching a funny movie, reading a captivating story, or listening to music that made our hearts sing. It was about allowing ourselves to be silly, to laugh until our bellies hurt, and to embrace the world with a child's wonder.

Sometimes, just spending time with family and friends, playing silly games or sharing stories, was enough to lift our spirits. The power of laughter and connection can be a magical cure, a balm for the soul.

Play wasn't a distraction from the reality of our situation; it was a way to embrace life, even in the midst of challenges. It was a reminder that even in the hospital, there was still space for joy, for wonder, for the magic of imagination. It was a way to keep our spirits high, to find strength within ourselves, and to face the ups and downs of treatment with a little more courage, a little more laughter, and a lot more hope.

KEEPING THE SPIRIT HIGH THROUGH CREATIVITY

Sometimes, the best way to chase away the shadows of fear and worry is to create our own sunshine. When I was in the hospital, surrounded by medical machines and the sterile smell of the place, it was easy to feel like I was trapped in a grey world. But I discovered that even in that world, I could paint my own colors. I had a magic box full of crayons and markers, and they were my secret weapons against the gloom.

Remember how I told you about the grumpy old IV pole in my room? Well, he wasn't so grumpy after all. He was just lonely, missing his adventures in the outside world. So, I decided to give him a makeover! With my colorful markers, I transformed him into a friendly robot. I named him "Iron Man" and we became the best of friends. He would watch over me while I slept, and I would tell him stories about my day.

The nurses loved Iron Man too. They would often stop by to chat with him, and I would proudly show them how I had decorated him with my own designs. It was a small thing, but it brought a little bit of laughter into the room, and it made me feel like I was in control, even though I was surrounded by so many things that I couldn't control.

My imagination also helped me to escape the hospital walls. When I was feeling tired or scared, I would close my eyes and imagine myself soaring through the sky with a flock of birds. Sometimes, I would imagine I was a brave explorer, discovering hidden treasures in a faraway land. These imaginary adventures helped me to forget about the needles and the tests, and they filled my heart with hope.

I even started making my own stories. They were silly stories, sometimes about talking animals or superheroes who lived in the hospital. My mom helped me write them down, and she would even illustrate them with pictures. We made a whole collection of "Hospital Adventures" stories, and I shared them with other kids in the ward. They loved them! And so did the doctors and nurses. It was a way for us all to connect and laugh together, even when things were tough.

One day, I decided to paint a mural on the wall of the playroom. It was a big mural, filled with colorful flowers, happy animals, and smiling children. It took me weeks to complete, but I was so proud of it when it was finished. The playroom was a lot brighter and more inviting with my mural, and it became a place where children could forget their worries and just have fun.

Painting the mural reminded me that even though I was going through a tough time, I could still make a difference. I could still bring joy to others, even if I was just a little kid in the hospital. And that's the thing about creativity; it reminds you that even in the darkest of times, you always have the power to choose light.

My art wasn't just a way to pass the time; it was a way to heal. It helped me to process my emotions, to express my fears and my hopes, and to find strength in myself..

I learned that when you're facing a challenge, it's important to find ways to make the world a little brighter, a little more beautiful, a little more filled with love.

I know that you are strong and brave, and you too can use creativity to overcome any obstacle. You might want to start with a drawing, a painting, a story, or a song. Whatever you choose, let your imagination soar and let your heart shine.

Who knows, maybe you will create something beautiful that will inspire others to face their own challenges with courage and resilience. I believe in you!

FINDING RESILIENCE IN EVERYDAY MOMENTS

Resilience isn't something you're born with, it's a muscle you build, a skill you cultivate. It's about finding those little sparks of strength within yourself, even on days when you feel like you're barely holding on. It's about recognizing that even the smallest victories, the little moments of joy, are worth celebrating. I remember those days in the hospital, when every step felt like a mountain to climb. I remember the endless tests, the pokes and prods, the fear that clung to me like a shadow. But even in the midst of that, I found glimmers of hope.

One day, while sitting in my room, I noticed a small, bright yellow butterfly fluttering outside my window. It seemed to be dancing on the wind, a tiny symbol of freedom and joy. I watched it for what felt like an eternity, and for those few moments, the fear and pain seemed to fade away. I felt a spark of hope, a reminder that beauty and light could still exist even in the darkest of times. That butterfly became a symbol for me, a reminder that even when everything feels overwhelming, there's always a reason to keep fighting.

I found resilience in the simplest of things: a warm hug from my mom, the sound of her voice reading me stories, the comforting silence of my dog sleeping beside me. I learned that love, in all its forms, was a powerful force, a source of strength that helped me weather the storms. And I found resilience in the small victories: a day when I felt strong enough to walk a little further, a day when I could eat a whole meal without feeling sick, a day when the nausea subsided just enough for me to laugh with my friends. Every little step forward, every moment of normalcy, was a victory worth celebrating.

One day, while sitting in the hospital waiting room, I noticed a young girl who was clearly struggling with her treatment. She was pale and tired, with a look of fear in her eyes. I remember feeling a pang of empathy, a connection to her struggles. But then I remembered my own journey, all the moments of resilience I had found within myself. I wanted to share that with her, to show her that even in the darkest of times, there was hope.

I walked over to her and smiled. "Hey," I said, "I know this is tough, but you're doing great. You're so strong." Her eyes widened in surprise, then softened into a small smile. We talked for a while, and I shared some of my own experiences, trying to show her that she wasn't alone. That small act of kindness, that moment of connection, was a reminder of the power of resilience. It wasn't just about my own strength; it was about sharing that strength with others, about showing them that they weren't alone in their struggles.

Resilience wasn't just about surviving; it was about thriving. It was about finding the joy in the little things, about embracing the unexpected, and about recognizing that even in the midst of hardship, there was always something to be grateful for. I remember feeling a sense of peace after finishing my treatment, a sense of accomplishment, knowing that I had faced my fears and come out stronger on the other side. But even more than that, I felt a deep sense of gratitude for all the people who had supported me, who had shown me kindness and love during my darkest times.

My experience taught me that resilience isn't about being strong all the time; it's about being vulnerable, about admitting when you need help, and about allowing yourself to be supported by others. It's about recognizing that even the smallest acts of kindness can have a profound impact, and that we are all connected in ways we may not always see.

Resilience is a journey, not a destination. It's a lifelong process of learning, adapting, and growing. It's about finding the strength within yourself, even when you feel like you've run out of steam. And most importantly, it's about never giving up hope, no matter how difficult things may seem.

I know this may all sound a little idealistic, but believe me, it's true. Resilience is real, and it's within all of us. We just have to learn how to tap into it. And once we do, we can face any challenge, overcome any obstacle, and emerge stronger on the other side. We can become beacons of hope, inspiring others to find their own inner strength and to embrace the journey, no matter how difficult it may be.

THE ROLE OF POSITIVITY AND OPTIMISM

The journey through cancer treatment can be a rollercoaster of emotions. One day you might be brimming with hope, feeling strong and optimistic about the future, while the next day might bring a wave of fear, fatigue, and uncertainty. It's during these challenging moments that the power of a positive mindset shines through. It's not about ignoring the difficulties or pretending everything is perfect. Instead, it's about actively choosing to focus on the good, finding reasons to smile, and believing in your body's ability to heal.

Imagine a tiny seed buried in the ground. It's dark, cold, and it might feel like nothing is happening. Yet, beneath the surface, the seed is drawing strength from the earth, absorbing nutrients, and preparing to grow. This seed represents our inner strength, the resilience we all possess. It might be hidden from view, but it's always there, waiting for the right conditions to bloom.

A positive mindset acts like sunshine and rain for that seed, providing the nourishment it needs to flourish. It's like a gentle nudge, reminding us that even when things feel tough, we have the power to choose hope. When we choose to see the good, to celebrate small victories, and to believe in our ability to overcome, we give that seed the strength it needs to grow.

Here's how a positive mindset can play a vital role in your healing journey:

1. Reducing Stress and Anxiety:

Cancer treatment can be physically and emotionally draining. There are appointments, tests, and procedures that can cause anxiety and fear. A positive outlook helps to manage these feelings. When you focus on the positive aspects of your life, your mind finds a sense of calm, reducing the overwhelming stress that can hinder your healing.

2. Strengthening the Immune System:

The immune system is our body's natural defense against illness. Studies have shown that a positive attitude can help strengthen the immune system, making it more effective in fighting off infections and promoting healing. By choosing to focus on positive thoughts, we send a message to our bodies to be strong and resilient.

3. Enhancing Pain Management:

Pain is a common side effect of cancer treatment. While medication plays an important role, a positive mindset can help you cope with pain more effectively. When you focus on positive thoughts, you distract your mind from the discomfort, making it easier to manage.

4. Fostering a Sense of Control:

Cancer can make you feel like you've lost control over your life. It can feel like everything is happening to you, leaving you feeling powerless. A positive mindset empowers you to take control of your healing journey. By focusing on what you can control - your attitude, your choices, your actions - you gain a sense of agency and empowerment, which can help you feel more confident in your ability to face challenges.

5. Building a Stronger Support Network:

A positive attitude can attract positive energy. People are drawn to those who radiate hope and optimism. When you approach your journey with a positive outlook, you inspire others to do the same. This creates a stronger support network around you, filled with people who offer encouragement, kindness, and compassion.

6. Discovering Hidden Strengths:

Cancer challenges you in ways you never imagined. It pushes you to dig deep within yourself and tap into reserves of strength you didn't know you had. A positive mindset allows you to see these strengths, to embrace them, and to use them as fuel to navigate the difficult moments. It helps you discover that you are stronger than you thought possible.

Finding Positivity in Everyday Moments:

A positive mindset doesn't mean ignoring the tough days. It's about finding the good even amidst challenges. It's about learning to appreciate the small things that bring you joy. Here are some ways to cultivate positivity in your daily life:

Gratitude Journal: Start a journal to write down things you are grateful for each day. It could be a delicious meal, a beautiful sunset, a kind word from a loved one, or simply the feeling of sunshine on your skin. **Mindful Moments:** Take a few moments each day to focus on your senses. Notice the colors, sounds, smells, and textures around you. This brings you back to the present moment and helps you appreciate the beauty of everyday life. **Acts of Kindness:** Do something nice for someone else, even something small. A smile, a helping hand, a thoughtful gesture can brighten someone's day and make you feel good.

Laughter is Medicine: Laughter is a powerful antidote to stress and negativity. Watch a funny movie, read a humorous book, or spend time with people who make you laugh.

Embrace the Little Things: Celebrate small victories, like finishing a meal, taking a walk, or having a good night's sleep. Each small step forward is a reason to be proud.

Remember, a positive mindset is not a magic cure. It doesn't erase the challenges or guarantee a perfect outcome. But it does give you the strength and resilience to navigate those challenges with hope and determination. It helps you find the courage to face each day, knowing that even in the darkest moments, there is always light within you.

Cultivating a Positive Mindset for Your Child:

If you are a parent or caregiver of a child going through cancer treatment, it's important to create a positive and supportive environment for them. Here are some tips:

Be Honest and Age-Appropriate: Explain what's happening in a way your child can understand, using simple and honest language. Avoid sugarcoating or hiding the truth.

Focus on the Positive: Talk about their strengths, their accomplishments, and the things they enjoy doing. Celebrate small victories, like finishing a treatment cycle or having a good day at school.

Encourage Creativity and Play: Allow them to express themselves through art, music, stories, or games. This helps them cope with their emotions and maintain a sense of normalcy.

Be a Source of Strength and Hope: Let your child know that you are there for them, no matter what. Offer your love, support, and reassurance.

Find Support for Yourself: Remember that you are not alone. Seek out support groups, online communities, or professional counseling to manage your own stress and emotions.

Sharing Your Story, Spreading Hope:

The experience of cancer can be transformative. It can change your perspective on life, making you more aware of the preciousness of each moment. When you share your story, you inspire others to find strength and hope. You become a beacon of light, guiding others through their own journeys.

Whether you're sharing your story with family, friends, a community group, or through writing, your words can have a profound impact. By sharing your challenges, your triumphs, and your lessons learned, you offer hope and encouragement to those who need it most.

You show others that even in the face of adversity, there is beauty, resilience, and hope. You remind everyone that even in the darkest of times, the human spirit can find a way to shine.

Remember, you are not alone. Your story is a powerful reminder that with strength, resilience, and a positive mindset, you can overcome any challenge. Embrace your journey, celebrate your victories, and never give up hope.

LEARNING FROM THE JOURNEY

The journey through cancer, while filled with challenges, is a transformative experience. It's a journey of self-discovery, where you learn about your inner strength and resilience, qualities that you may not have known you possessed. It's a journey of self-acceptance, where you learn to embrace the beauty of your vulnerability and the power of seeking support from others. It's a journey of gratitude, where you learn to appreciate the simple joys of life and the beauty of human connection.

As I navigated through my own cancer experience, I discovered that while the journey was filled with fear and uncertainty, it also offered opportunities for growth and profound self-reflection. Every day was a lesson, every challenge a chance to find strength. The journey taught me the value of hope, the importance of building a strong support network, and the power of a positive mindset. I learned to embrace the ups and downs of treatment, to celebrate the small victories, and to find joy in the ordinary moments.

One of the most profound lessons I learned was the importance of embracing vulnerability. It's okay to be afraid, to feel overwhelmed, to need support. Allowing myself to be vulnerable allowed me to connect with others, to share my journey, and to receive the love and support I needed. It helped me break down the walls I had built around myself, fostering a deeper understanding and appreciation of my own needs and emotions.

Through the challenges of treatment, I discovered an incredible strength within myself. I learned that I could face any obstacle with courage and determination, that I could handle adversity with grace, and that I could find joy even in the midst of pain. The fight for survival became a fight for self-discovery, a journey of inner exploration, where I unearthed a reservoir of strength I didn't know existed.

The journey also taught me the power of hope. It taught me that even when things seem darkest, there is always light at the end of the tunnel. It taught me to hold on to the belief that even when facing the impossible, there is always hope for a better tomorrow. The journey taught me to find hope in the small things, in the smiles of loved ones, in the beauty of nature, in the simple act of being alive.

I learned to appreciate the importance of building a strong support network. I learned that I was not alone in this fight and that I had people who cared about me, who were there to support me every step of the way. I learned to lean on my family, my friends, and even strangers who offered their kindness and compassion. I learned the value of shared experiences, of knowing that others had walked a similar path and understood my struggles.

The journey taught me the importance of a positive mindset. I learned that thoughts have power, that our minds can influence our bodies, and that we can choose to focus on the positive even when faced with negativity. I learned to use my imagination to create a world of hope, a world where I could see myself getting better, a world where I could envision a future filled with joy and possibility.

The experience of surviving cancer has given me a new perspective on life. It has made me appreciate the simple joys of life, the beauty of human connection, and the preciousness of every moment. It has made me more compassionate, more understanding, and more grateful for the gift of life.

My journey through cancer taught me that strength comes not from being fearless, but from facing your fears with courage and determination. It taught me that resilience is not about avoiding pain, but about finding ways to navigate it and come out stronger on the other side. It taught me that hope is not a wishful thought, but a powerful force that can guide us through even the darkest times.

The journey taught me that I am stronger than I thought I was, that I have the capacity to overcome any obstacle, that I am capable of finding joy even in the face of hardship, and that I have the power to create a life filled with purpose and meaning.

It is my hope that by sharing my story, I can empower others who are facing similar challenges. I want to offer hope, encouragement, and a reminder that they are not alone. I want to inspire them to find their inner strength, to embrace their vulnerability, to cultivate a positive mindset, and to believe in the power of hope.

The journey through cancer is not easy, but it can be a journey of self-discovery, growth, and resilience. It can be a journey that teaches us about our own inner strength, the importance of human connection, and the power of hope. It can be a journey that transforms us, leaving us stronger, wiser, and more grateful for the gift of life.

EMPOWERING OTHERS THROUGH MY STORY

The most rewarding part of my journey wasn't just surviving cancer, but finding ways to help others navigate their own battles. Sharing my story became a way to light a path for those who needed it most. It was a chance to offer comfort, strength, and the hope that even in the darkest moments, there is always light.

As I began speaking at schools, hospitals, and community events, I realized the profound impact of my words. I saw it in the wide eyes of children who had never encountered cancer before, in the hopeful smiles of those battling their own diagnoses, and in the tearful nods of parents who were seeking answers and solace. My story became a bridge between their fears and my own experiences, a reminder that they weren't alone in this fight.

I learned that vulnerability is strength. It takes courage to share your deepest fears and triumphs, to lay bare the raw emotions that accompany a cancer diagnosis. Yet, in doing so, I connected with others in a way that I never thought possible. They saw themselves in my journey, they felt my pain, and they embraced my strength. They understood that fear and uncertainty are natural parts of the process, but they also witnessed how love, support, and an unwavering belief in one's own resilience could guide them through.

One of the most impactful moments I experienced occurred at a local school. The principal had invited me to speak to a group of fourth-grade students. As I shared my story, I noticed a young girl in the front row with tears streaming down her face. After my talk, she approached me with trembling hands. She told me she had a friend who was battling leukemia, and she was terrified. I listened intently, my heart aching for her friend and her own fear. I told her that I understood, that I had felt the same way, but that she wasn't alone.

I shared how I had found strength in the love of my family and friends, in the kindness of strangers, and in the unwavering support of the medical team. I emphasized the importance of hope, of dreaming big, and of believing in the possibility of a brighter future. As we spoke, the girl's tears subsided, replaced by a glimmer of hope. She left that day with a renewed sense of courage and the knowledge that she wasn't facing this alone.

Sharing my story wasn't about making light of the struggles or pretending that cancer is easy. It was about honesty, about acknowledging the challenges and embracing the lessons learned along the way. It was about offering a hand to those walking the same path, a shoulder to lean on during the hardest moments, and a voice of hope when the world seemed to fade away.

This wasn't just about survival; it was about thriving. It was about demonstrating that even in the face of adversity, the human spirit is capable of incredible strength and resilience. It was about empowering others to find their own inner warrior, to tap into the vast reserves of courage that lie within each of us.

Every time I shared my story, I received more than I gave. I gained new perspectives, deepened my own understanding, and discovered a purpose beyond my own healing. I learned that true strength lies not in overcoming the odds, but in using our experiences to uplift others, to inspire them to rise above their challenges, and to embrace life with a newfound appreciation for its preciousness.

The impact of sharing my story extended far beyond the individuals I spoke to. It inspired others to contribute to cancer research, to volunteer their time at hospitals, and to show acts of kindness to those in need. It ignited a chain reaction of compassion and empathy, proving that even the smallest act of support can make a world of difference.

Sharing my story wasn't just about me; it was about all of us. It was about connecting with each other, sharing our experiences, and recognizing the universal human desire for strength, hope, and healing. It was a reminder that we are all interconnected, and that in our shared vulnerability, we find our greatest strength. And that is a message worth sharing with the world.

THE POWER OF HOPE
AND DREAMS

Hope, like a tiny, flickering flame, danced in the depths of my heart, refusing to be extinguished by the storm of fear and uncertainty that raged around me. It was a whisper in the silence, a ray of sunshine piercing through the clouds of despair. It was the belief that even in the darkest of times, there was still light to be found, a possibility of a future, a chance to see the world anew.

Hope was the anchor that kept me tethered to the present, even when the future felt like a distant, blurry dream. It was the unwavering belief that this journey, however arduous, would eventually lead to a destination of healing and growth. It was the courage to face the unknown, to trust in the power of time and the resilience of the human spirit.

Hope, however, was not a passive emotion, a mere wishful thinking. It was an active force, a constant companion on this extraordinary journey. It was the spark that ignited my determination to fight, to embrace each day with a newfound appreciation for life's simple joys. It was the fuel that propelled me forward, urging me to seek out every opportunity to find strength within myself and around me.

Hope was the source of my dreams, the seeds of possibility planted deep within my heart. It was the vision of a future filled with laughter, adventure, and boundless possibilities. It was the dream of playing with my friends, of dancing in the rain, of exploring the world with eyes wide open. It was the desire to live a full, meaningful life, a life where the scars of this journey would serve as reminders of my inner strength and the unwavering spirit that had carried me through.

Hope, like a beautiful butterfly, gently guided me through the labyrinth of treatment, reminding me that even in the midst of challenges, there was always beauty to be found. It was the delicate wings that carried me through the toughest of days, whispering words of encouragement and reminding me of my inherent worth.

In the hospital room, surrounded by sterile walls and the hum of machines, hope would often take the form of a simple, playful melody, sung by a beloved family member. It was the warmth of a hug, the gentle touch of a friend's hand, the laughter of a child. It was the stories shared, the memories cherished, the moments of joy that punctuated the somber days.

Hope was also found in the unexpected places, the moments of kindness that appeared like stars in the darkest night. It was the smile of a stranger, the compassionate words of a nurse, the generosity of a community that rallied around me. It was the feeling of being loved, supported, and understood, a feeling that sustained me through every challenge.

Hope, like a compass, guided me toward my goals, reminding me that the journey was not just about surviving, but about thriving. It was the belief that I was capable of exceeding my own expectations, of rising above the limitations imposed by the illness. It was the courage to dream big, to envision a future filled with possibilities, a future where I could make a difference in the world.

Hope was the promise of a brighter tomorrow, a future where I could finally see the world through eyes free from the burden of illness. It was the anticipation of experiencing life to the fullest, of discovering my passions, of pursuing my dreams with unwavering zeal. It was the belief that this journey, although painful, would ultimately lead to a life filled with purpose, meaning, and joy.

Hope was not simply a wish, but a powerful tool that fueled my resilience and guided me toward a future filled with possibilities. It was the strength that propelled me forward, reminding me that even in the face of adversity, there was always hope for a brighter tomorrow. It was the belief that I could not only survive this journey, but thrive and inspire others along the way.

ADAPTING TO A NEW NORMAL

The hospital room felt different now. The whirring of machines and the constant buzz of activity had faded into a soft hum. The sterile white walls, once a constant reminder of my illness, now felt a bit more welcoming. It was time to go home.

The journey back to my life was a new adventure, a whole new set of feelings I was trying to navigate. The fear of the unknown lingered, a shadow at the edges of my thoughts. Would I be different now? Would my body ever feel like it used to? Would everyone look at me differently?

At first, going back to school was like stepping into a dream. Everything felt a little blurry, the familiar faces slightly out of focus. The classroom seemed smaller, the playground seemed quieter. It was as if I had been gone for a very long time, even though it had only been a few months.

The other children seemed to know how to navigate this space, how to move through the world with ease. I, on the other hand, felt clumsy, uncertain, like I was learning to walk all over again. The laughter, the whispers, the glances felt like a kaleidoscope of emotions swirling around me. It was overwhelming, a tidal wave of sensations I wasn't sure how to handle.

But then, a familiar hand reached out, pulling me into the familiar rhythm of the school day. My best friend, Sarah, with her bright smile and her infectious laughter, helped me find my way back to my old world. She explained things I had missed, shared jokes, and patiently listened to my anxieties.

"It's going to be okay," she said, her voice filled with a quiet confidence that soothed my fears. "It's just going to take a little time."

And it did. Slowly, bit by bit, I found my way back to the familiar rhythm of my life. I started to participate in school activities again, enjoying the games, the laughter, and the camaraderie of my friends. The fear that had haunted me began to fade, replaced by a sense of cautious optimism.

But some things had changed. The world looked a little different now, with a new appreciation for its simple joys. I noticed the sunlight dappling through the trees, the warmth of the sun on my skin, the laughter of children playing in the park. Before, these things had been just everyday occurrences, a backdrop to my life. Now, they felt like gifts, small miracles I was grateful to experience.

The world had always been full of color, but now I saw it in a new light. The vibrant green of the leaves, the deep blue of the sky, the bright yellow of the sunflowers seemed to have a new vibrancy, as if the world itself was celebrating my return.

Sometimes, the memories of the hospital would creep in, like a wisp of smoke, reminding me of the journey I had been through. The needles, the tests, the long nights filled with fear, the constant weariness. But these memories were no longer tinged with fear, but with a sense of pride and resilience. I had fought and survived, and I had learned so much along the way.

I had learned about the strength within me, a wellspring of courage I never knew I possessed. I had learned about the power of hope, the ability to believe in the possibility of healing, even when it seemed impossible. I had learned about the love and support of family and friends, the unwavering bond that carried me through the darkest days.

The journey hadn't been easy, but it had changed me. It had made me stronger, more compassionate, more grateful. I had found a new appreciation for life, a deeper understanding of its fragility and its beauty.

Life after cancer was not the same, but it was a beautiful new normal. I had learned to embrace the changes, the challenges, the triumphs. I had found a new rhythm, a new appreciation for the world around me, and a new strength within myself. The journey had taken me through a storm, but it had also revealed a clear, bright sky, full of possibilities.

The future was still unknown, but I knew that with each step I took, with each new experience I embraced, I was writing a new story, a story of resilience, hope, and love. The journey had been long and challenging, but the end result was a story of triumph, a reminder that even in the face of adversity, life finds a way to bloom.

NEW PERSPECTIVES AND GRATITUDE

The hospital walls, once so sterile and intimidating, now felt like familiar companions. The beeping machines, the scent of antiseptic, and the hushed whispers of nurses – these were the sounds and smells of my new reality. I had been through so much in the past few months, yet there was a growing sense of gratitude that had settled deep within me.

Before cancer, life was a blur of school, friends, and playdates. I took things for granted, not realizing the preciousness of each passing moment. Now, with every sunrise, I woke up with a profound appreciation for the simple joys that I had once overlooked.

The sunbeams filtering through the window, casting dancing shadows on the hospital room floor, now held a magic I had never noticed before. The familiar chirping of birds outside, once just background noise, now filled my heart with an unexpected joy. The warmth of my mother's hand in mine, and the laughter of my siblings – these were the anchors that kept me grounded during the storm.

Even the smallest things became beacons of hope. The brightly colored flowers that my friends sent, the funny cartoons my doctor drew on my chart, the silly jokes that nurses shared to lighten the mood – they all reminded me that even in the face of hardship, there was still beauty and kindness in the world.

Each day, I felt a shift within me. The fear that had once consumed me began to dissipate, replaced by a newfound strength. The doctors and nurses, who I had initially perceived as figures of authority, transformed into trusted allies. Their expertise, their compassion, and their unwavering support filled me with a sense of security and trust.

There were moments of despair, moments when the exhaustion and the side effects of treatment overwhelmed me. But even in those moments, I learned to find solace in the little things.

I would escape into the world of books, letting the stories transport me to other places, far away from the sterile hospital walls. I would draw pictures, using my imagination to create worlds filled with vibrant colors and fantastical creatures. I would listen to music, letting the melodies wash over me, calming my anxieties and reminding me of the beauty that still existed.

These simple acts, these tiny moments of joy, helped me to weather the storms. They reminded me that even in the darkest of times, there was always a flicker of hope, a reason to keep fighting.

The experience of cancer forced me to confront my mortality, to confront my own limitations. But it also opened my eyes to the beauty of life, to the strength of the human spirit, and to the power of love and connection.

I learned that true happiness wasn't found in material possessions or external validation, but in the simple act of being present, of appreciating the beauty around me, and of cherishing the bonds I shared with those I loved.

Cancer, in its cruel irony, had become a catalyst for growth. It had stripped me bare, exposing my vulnerabilities, but it had also allowed me to rediscover my inner strength, to redefine what it meant to be truly alive.

Life after cancer was not about erasing the past or forgetting the pain. It was about embracing the lessons learned, about carrying the scars of my journey with pride, and about living each day with an unwavering sense of gratitude. I had walked through the valley of shadows, but I had emerged stronger, more resilient, and more alive than ever before.

This newfound appreciation for life extended beyond my own experiences. I found myself noticing the simple joys in the lives of others, the laughter of children playing, the warmth of a stranger's smile, the kindness of a helping hand. I felt a deep sense of empathy for those who were facing their own challenges, and I wanted to share the lessons I had learned, to offer a glimmer of hope, and to remind them that even in the darkest of times, there was always light to be found.

The world felt more vibrant, more alive, and more meaningful than ever before. I was no longer simply existing; I was truly living, embracing every moment, every breath, every sunrise, and every sunset with a newfound appreciation for the precious gift of life. And I knew, with absolute certainty, that my journey had just begun.

THE STRENGTH IN VULNERABILITY

The world felt different now. It wasn't just the hospital walls and the constant beeping of machines that made me feel uneasy. It was something deeper, a sense of vulnerability that I hadn't known before. The days of carefree laughter and boundless energy were replaced with a quiet stillness, a cautious awareness of my own fragility.

I remember one particular day, sitting in the sterile white room, a blanket wrapped around me like a shield against the cold. The doctor, a kind woman with eyes that held a mixture of concern and hope, explained the latest test results. It wasn't the words she spoke, but the way she paused, her voice softening as she gently placed her hand on mine.

"This is a lot to take in, sweetheart," she said, her touch surprisingly reassuring. "It's okay to feel scared, to feel overwhelmed. It's a part of the journey."

Her words, so simple yet profound, resonated deep within me. For the first time, I understood that vulnerability wasn't weakness. It was the space between the fear and the hope, where honesty and acceptance could flourish. It was the courage to acknowledge my limitations, my anxieties, and my need for support.

It was in that moment of vulnerability that I found a new strength. A strength that came not from pushing away my emotions, but from embracing them. A strength that allowed me to lean on my family, my friends, and even the strangers who had become my companions in this unexpected adventure.

The days that followed were still filled with challenges, with moments of doubt and fear. But I knew, deep down, that it was okay to feel those emotions. It was okay to be vulnerable. It was in that vulnerability that I discovered a new kind of bravery, a bravery that came from accepting my limitations and finding strength in the support of others.

I learned that vulnerability wasn't a sign of weakness, but a source of connection. It was the bridge that allowed me to reach out, to ask for help, to share my fears and my hopes. It was the key that unlocked a network of support that I didn't even know existed.

One day, while I was sitting in the waiting area, I noticed a young girl with a bright smile, playing with a toy spaceship. Her eyes were filled with a quiet determination that reminded me of myself. She was battling a different kind of cancer, but her spirit was as strong as mine.

I watched as she interacted with other patients, offering them a smile, a kind word, a simple gesture of empathy. It was a reminder that even in the face of fear and uncertainty, we could find the strength to connect with others, to share our experiences, and to offer comfort and encouragement.

That day, I decided to share my own story with her. I told her about my journey, about the challenges and triumphs, about the vulnerability and the strength I had found.

"It's okay to feel scared," I told her, "but don't let fear hold you back. Find your strength in the people who love you, in the moments of joy, in the simple things that make you smile."

Her eyes widened, her smile growing brighter. "You're brave," she said, "and you're helping me to be brave too."

In that moment, I understood the true power of vulnerability. It wasn't just about sharing our own struggles, but about reaching out to others, offering them a hand, a listening ear, a kind word. It was about creating a space of shared experiences, where we could learn from each other, support each other, and find strength in the collective embrace of humanity.

The journey of healing is a long and winding road, filled with twists and turns, moments of joy and sorrow, days of triumph and moments of doubt. It's a journey that tests our resilience, pushes our limits, and ultimately, reveals the depths of our strength. But it's also a journey that invites us to embrace vulnerability, to acknowledge our limitations, and to find solace in the bonds of connection.

It's in the shared vulnerability that we discover the true meaning of courage, the power of hope, and the unwavering strength of the human spirit. It's in those moments of vulnerability that we learn to appreciate the beauty of life, the resilience of the human spirit, and the transformative power of connection. And in that journey, we discover that vulnerability is not a sign of weakness, but a source of strength, a bridge to connection, and a testament to the beauty of the human spirit.

BUILDING NEW DREAMS AND GOALS

The hospital walls were no longer just walls. They were canvases painted with stories, each crack and chip telling a tale of courage and resilience. The machines hummed like a symphony of hope, their mechanical sounds a familiar lullaby now. It was a world I knew intimately, a world that had become a part of me. But as the final treatment drew near, a new kind of excitement began to stir within. The excitement of a new adventure, a chapter about to be written – a chapter about the future.

The future. It was a word that had once been tinged with uncertainty, a word that whispered of the unknown. But now, it held the promise of possibility, a blank canvas waiting to be filled with dreams and aspirations. It was the future that I, with newfound courage and a heart overflowing with gratitude, was ready to embrace.

The journey to this point had been arduous, filled with moments of despair and doubt. But it had also taught me the power of perseverance, the strength that lies within, and the boundless love that surrounds us. I had learned to appreciate the small victories – the ringing of the hospital bell signaling the end of a treatment cycle, the laughter shared with newfound friends in the playroom, the joy of simply waking up each morning.

Now, as the final chapter of my cancer story neared its close, I was ready to rewrite the narrative. I was ready to write a story of hope, a story of dreams, a story of building a life filled with purpose and meaning.

The world outside the hospital walls beckoned. It was a world waiting to be explored, a world that held endless possibilities. The whispers of doubt and fear that had haunted my thoughts during treatment were now replaced by a chorus of optimism and anticipation. I had faced the darkness and emerged into the light, and in doing so, I had discovered a strength within myself that I never knew existed.

What did I want to do with this newfound freedom? The answer was simple: I wanted to live, I wanted to love, I wanted to dream big. I wanted to explore the world with the same boundless curiosity I had as a child, but with the added wisdom and resilience that my journey had bestowed upon me.

I envisioned a life filled with laughter, with adventure, with purpose. I imagined myself pursuing passions I had long put on hold, learning new skills, embracing new challenges, and making a difference in the world.

I knew there would be hurdles to overcome, there would be days of doubt and fear, but I also knew that I was equipped with the tools to navigate them. I had faced the unimaginable, and I had come out stronger on the other side. I had learned to embrace the unexpected, to find beauty in the ordinary, and to believe in the power of my own resilience.

The future was no longer an empty canvas; it was a landscape teeming with possibility. It was a landscape I was determined to explore, a landscape I was ready to shape with my own hands.

The thought of a future filled with dreams and aspirations filled me with a sense of awe and excitement. I wanted to travel the world, to experience different cultures, to learn new languages. I wanted to write stories that would inspire and uplift, to create art that would move hearts and minds.

And I knew, with absolute certainty, that I would. I had tasted the bitter sting of loss, the fear of the unknown, the pain of vulnerability. But I had also tasted the sweetness of victory, the joy of connection, the power of hope. And in that knowledge, I found the strength to dream.

The future was mine to create. It was a blank canvas waiting for me to paint my own masterpiece. And as I embarked on this new journey, I knew that I was not alone. I had a support system that was unwavering, a community that believed in me, and a spirit that was unyielding.

I was a survivor. And I was ready to thrive.

The dreams I held close to my heart were not just for me. They were for the children who were fighting their own battles, for the families who were walking beside them, for the world that needed hope and inspiration.

My journey had taught me that every single one of us has the power to overcome adversity, to find strength in our vulnerabilities, and to dream big, no matter what life throws our way.

And so, I set out to build my new dreams, brick by brick, with every step forward, with every challenge faced, with every victory celebrated. I knew that the path ahead would not always be easy, but I also knew that I was capable of anything, that I was worthy of a life filled with joy, with purpose, with dreams that were both grand and deeply personal.

The cancer journey was a journey of change and growth, a journey that had transformed me in ways I could never have imagined. It had stripped away my fears, my insecurities, my need for control. It had shown me the true meaning of courage, of resilience, of hope.

And now, as I stood on the precipice of a new chapter, I was ready to embrace the change, to welcome the growth, to build a life that was truly my own.

I was a cancer survivor. And I was ready to create a future filled with dreams, a future filled with love, a future filled with the unwavering belief that anything is possible.

A LOOK BACK AT
THE JOURNEY

The journey was a whirlwind of emotions, a rollercoaster ride that took me from the depths of fear to the heights of hope. It was a testament to the resilience of the human spirit, a reminder that even in the darkest of times, there is always a flicker of light. It taught me the true meaning of strength, not just the physical kind but the kind that comes from within, the kind that allows you to face challenges head-on and emerge stronger on the other side.

Looking back, I am filled with a sense of gratitude. Gratitude for the unwavering support of my family, the love and encouragement of my friends, and the dedication of the medical professionals who fought alongside me. I am grateful for the lessons I learned, the strength I discovered, and the newfound appreciation for the simple joys of life.

The road to recovery was not easy. There were moments of doubt, fear, and exhaustion. But there were also moments of triumph, resilience, and hope. Each treatment, each hurdle overcome, was a victory in itself. It was during these moments of struggle and triumph that I realized the true meaning of bravery. It wasn't about being fearless, but about facing my fears with courage and determination.

My cancer journey wasn't just about me. It was about the people around me, the love they showered upon me, and the lessons I learned from them. My mother, my rock, my constant source of strength, showed me the meaning of unconditional love and unwavering support. My siblings, my playmates, my constant source of laughter, taught me the importance of family and the power of a shared smile. My friends, my confidantes, my constant source of encouragement, reminded me that I was not alone in this journey.

The hospital became my second home, a place filled with both joy and sorrow. I met other children who were battling their own personal battles, each facing their own unique challenges. In their eyes, I saw the same fear, the same hope, the same desire to get better. We shared our stories, our fears, and our dreams, creating a bond of shared experience. These encounters taught me the power of empathy, the importance of compassion, and the beauty of human connection.

The treatment was grueling, physically and emotionally draining. There were days when I felt weak and tired, days when I questioned my strength, days when I simply wanted to give up. But then, I would remember the faces of my loved ones, their smiles, their unwavering belief in me, and I would find the courage to push forward.

I learned to appreciate the small things, the simple joys that had once been taken for granted. A warm hug from my mother, a silly joke from my brother, the taste of my favorite ice cream, the laughter of my friends – these were the moments that filled my days with happiness and reminded me that life was worth fighting for.

My journey was a constant process of learning, a constant exploration of my inner strength. I learned to navigate the complexities of treatment, to manage the physical and emotional challenges, and to find joy in the midst of adversity. I learned the importance of communication, the power of laughter, and the healing touch of love.

I learned that courage is not the absence of fear, but the ability to act despite it. I learned that resilience is not about being tough, but about being adaptable and finding ways to bounce back from adversity. I learned that hope is not a passive dream, but an active force that fuels our spirit and guides our path.

The impact of my journey was profound. It reshaped my perspective on life, deepened my appreciation for the people around me, and instilled in me a sense of purpose. I realized that my story had the potential to empower others, to inspire hope, and to provide a sense of comfort to those facing similar challenges.

I discovered a passion for sharing my story, for using my experience to make a difference in the lives of others. I became a motivational speaker, sharing my journey with children battling cancer and their families, offering words of encouragement, and reminding them that they are not alone.

My journey taught me that even in the face of adversity, there is always hope. It taught me that strength comes from within, that love is the greatest healer, and that life is a precious gift to be cherished. It taught me that we are all capable of amazing things, that we are all stronger than we think, and that even the smallest act of kindness can make a world of difference.

As I look back on my journey, I am filled with a sense of gratitude, a sense of purpose, and a deep sense of hope for the future. My journey is a testament to the resilience of the human spirit, a reminder that even in the darkest of times, there is always light to be found. It is a story of courage, resilience, and hope, a story that I am proud to share with the world.

BECOMING A BEACON FOR OTHERS

The journey through cancer is a deeply personal one, but it's also a shared experience. As I looked back on my own fight, I realized that the strength and hope I had found wasn't just for myself, but for others facing the same challenges. I wanted to share my story, not just as a survivor, but as a beacon of hope for those who felt lost and scared.

I understood that sharing a story wasn't enough. People needed guidance, tools, and a sense of community to navigate their own battles. So, I began to think about how I could best support others, not just with words, but with tangible actions.

One of the most impactful things I learned during my treatment was the power of connection. Sharing my experiences with other patients and their families helped me feel less alone. I realized that hearing stories of resilience, of finding joy in the midst of hardship, and of the unwavering support of loved ones, offered a lifeline of hope.

I wanted to create a space where people could connect, share their struggles, and find comfort in knowing they weren't alone. I envisioned a community where stories of courage, resilience, and hope could be shared, inspiring and empowering others.

Building a supportive community was a crucial step in my journey to become a beacon for others. I started small, reaching out to fellow survivors, sharing my story, and offering a listening ear. I joined online forums, participated in support groups, and even created a small website where people could share their experiences.

These platforms became safe spaces for people to express their emotions, ask questions, and find solace in shared experiences. I learned that listening without judgment, offering encouragement, and sharing resources could make a world of difference in someone's life.

I also recognized the importance of raising awareness and educating others about cancer. I began giving talks at schools, hospitals, and community centers, sharing my story in a way that was relatable and inspiring to young audiences. I spoke about the importance of early detection, the power of positivity, and the strength that comes from seeking support.

My goal was to break down the stigma surrounding cancer, to show that even in the face of hardship, life can be filled with joy, love, and hope. I wanted to empower children to understand that they weren't alone in their battles, that there was a community of support waiting for them.

It wasn't always easy. There were times when I felt overwhelmed by the responsibility of sharing my story and offering support to others. But the joy and gratitude I saw in the eyes of those I connected with fueled my determination.

I also realized that my journey wasn't just about my own recovery, but about the legacy I could leave behind. I wanted to create a ripple effect of hope, inspiring others to find strength within themselves and to extend that same kindness and support to others in need.

I started to see the impact of my efforts in the lives of those I touched. Children who once felt scared and alone started to see their own journeys with new perspectives. Families found strength in knowing that they weren't facing this alone. And communities came together to support each other in ways they never imagined.

My journey taught me that the power of hope and resilience is contagious. By sharing my story and creating a community of support, I realized that I wasn't just helping others, I was also helping myself. The act of giving back brought a sense of purpose and meaning to my life.

I learned that even though the journey through cancer can be dark and challenging, it can also be a catalyst for personal growth, compassion, and a deeper understanding of what it means to be human. The light of hope, once ignited, can illuminate the path for others, leaving a legacy of strength and resilience that lasts far beyond our own struggles.

CREATING A SUPPORTIVE COMMUNITY

The journey through cancer is a solitary one, yet it doesn't have to be. The road ahead can be paved with strength and resilience, but also with the unwavering support of a loving community. This community, which we so carefully nurture, becomes our haven, a place where we find solace, understanding, and the courage to face our fears. It's a tapestry woven from the threads of shared experiences, kind words, and compassionate hearts.

Imagine a young girl named Lily, diagnosed with a Wilms tumor. The world around her seems to shrink, her fears and anxieties growing larger by the day. But then, a comforting warmth envelops her - her family, her friends, and the strangers who have become her newfound allies. Her parents become her unwavering pillars of support, their love a beacon in the storm. Their presence, their gentle touch, and their words of encouragement provide a safe haven for her fragile heart.

Lily's journey takes her to the hospital, a place that initially feels daunting and unfamiliar. But within these sterile walls, a new kind of community emerges. The other children battling their own challenges, their faces etched with bravery, become her comrades. They share their laughter, their fears, their stories of resilience. They bond over shared experiences, understanding the silent language of courage and hope. They share games, stories, and laughter, creating a space where the walls of fear crumble and a sense of camaraderie blooms.

The support doesn't stop at the hospital walls. Lily's school friends, their voices echoing through letters and messages, become a constant reminder of the world outside. These tokens of love and encouragement fuel her spirit, reminding her that she is not alone in her journey. They send drawings, jokes, and words of comfort, weaving a virtual tapestry of love and support that strengthens her resolve.

Beyond the individual connections, Lily finds solace in the community rallying around her. Local businesses organize fundraising events, offering a tangible expression of their support. The community comes together, their hearts filled with compassion and a desire to make a difference. The outpouring of love, the warm smiles, and the collective effort to ease her burden become a beacon of hope. Lily feels seen, heard, and cherished, her heart filled with gratitude for the generosity of those around her.

Even her furry companions, her loyal pets, contribute to the tapestry of her support system. They are a constant source of unconditional love and comfort, their presence providing a sense of peace and normalcy in the midst of chaos. Their warm bodies, their playful antics, and their silent companionship ease her anxieties and remind her of the simple joys that life has to offer.

Building a supportive community is not a passive act; it's an active choice, a deliberate effort to create a network of love and understanding. It's about reaching out, extending a hand of friendship, and offering a listening ear. It's about sharing burdens and celebrating victories, weaving a tapestry of shared experiences that binds us together.

For Lily, this community becomes her armor, her shield, and her source of strength. It reminds her that even in the darkest of times, she is not alone. It empowers her to face her fears, to embrace her vulnerability, and to emerge stronger and more resilient on the other side.

The power of community transcends the individual journey. It inspires others to reach out, to offer support, and to create a world where kindness and compassion are the norm. It's a testament to the human spirit's ability to overcome adversity, to find solace in shared experiences, and to create a legacy of hope for future generations.

This journey, though challenging, is a reminder that we are not meant to navigate it alone. We are woven into a tapestry of love, support, and resilience, a tapestry that extends beyond the individual and embraces the collective human spirit. And within this tapestry, we find the courage to face our fears, to embrace our vulnerabilities, and to emerge stronger and more resilient on the other side.

THE IMPACT OF KINDNESS AND COMPASSION

Kindness, like a warm embrace on a chilly day, has the power to soothe the soul and mend the spirit. It's a universal language that transcends words, whispering comfort and understanding in moments of vulnerability. Throughout my own cancer journey, I discovered the immense impact of kindness, both as a recipient and a giver. It was a constant source of strength, a beacon of light in the darkest of times.

The kindness I experienced started right at home. My mother , with her unwavering love and support, was my rock. She held my hand through every procedure, explained complex medical terms in simple ways, and never let me doubt her belief in my strength. She showered me with love, laughter, and countless cuddles, reminding me that I was not alone.

Beyond my family, the hospital walls became a tapestry woven with threads of compassion. The nurses, with their gentle touch and reassuring smiles, made the sterile environment feel a bit more human. They listened to my fears and anxieties, offering comfort and understanding without judgment. They treated me not just as a patient but as a person, recognizing my individuality and spirit.

One day, a young volunteer named Sarah brought me a handmade doll. It was crafted with meticulous detail, its delicate features resembling a princess from my favorite fairytale. Sarah, with her quiet grace and infectious smile, spent hours with me, reading stories and sharing her own experiences. Her simple act of kindness, her willingness to connect with me on a personal level, made a profound difference.

I learned that kindness doesn't always come from grand gestures or public displays. Often, it's found in the quiet moments, the small acts of love that resonate deeply. It was in the card from my best friend, penned with heartfelt words of encouragement, that reminded me of the world outside the hospital walls. It was in the warm smile of a fellow patient's parent, who offered a comforting word during a particularly challenging day. These moments of kindness, like tiny sparks, ignited a flame of hope within me.

But the impact of kindness wasn't a one-way street. I found that giving back, extending a helping hand to others, brought me a sense of purpose and fulfillment that transcended my own struggles. I started by sharing my story with other children going through similar experiences. I spoke about my fears and anxieties, but also about my strength, my determination, and the unwavering support that had sustained me.

I realized that vulnerability, far from being a weakness, was a source of strength. Sharing my story allowed me to connect with others, build a community of support, and offer a glimmer of hope to those facing similar challenges. It was a reminder that we're all in this together, that our shared experiences have the power to unite us.

One afternoon, I met a young girl named Emily, who was grappling with her own diagnosis. She was scared, confused, and overwhelmed. Her eyes, filled with fear, mirrored my own from years ago. I saw myself in her, and I knew I had to reach out.

I shared my story with Emily, focusing on the positive moments, the laughter, the joy, the love, and the resilience. I spoke about the strength within her, the beauty of life, and the power of hope. As I shared, I saw a flicker of recognition in her eyes, a spark of hope igniting within her.

In that moment, I realized that kindness wasn't just about receiving; it was about giving back, spreading the light of hope, and reminding others that they were not alone. It was about creating a ripple effect, a chain reaction of compassion that would touch countless lives.

The journey through cancer was arduous, filled with challenges and uncertainties. But it was kindness, the unwavering support of loved ones, the compassion of strangers, and the power of sharing my story that illuminated the path and strengthened my spirit. It was a journey that taught me the true meaning of resilience, the power of human connection, and the transformative impact of kindness.

As I navigate life after cancer, I carry the lessons learned with me. I continue to share my story, offering hope and inspiration to others. I strive to extend kindness and compassion to those in need, knowing that even the smallest act can make a world of difference. For in a world often filled with darkness, kindness is the light that guides us, the warmth that comforts us, and the strength that empowers us to overcome even the most challenging of journeys.

THE LEGACY OF COURAGE AND RESILIENCE

The legacy of courage and resilience I carry is not just mine; it's a torch I've been entrusted to pass on. This is the essence of sharing the light of hope – to illuminate the path for others who might find themselves in similar situations. Every time I share my story, I plant a seed of hope in the hearts of others. I believe that the power of one person's experience can create ripples of courage and inspire others to face their own challenges with strength and determination.

One of the most profound ways I can leave a legacy is by creating a supportive community. This isn't just about building networks and support groups; it's about fostering a sense of belonging, understanding, and shared purpose. It's about creating spaces where people can connect, share their experiences, and find solace in knowing they're not alone. I strive to create these spaces in my own life – through online forums, local events, and personal connections – where individuals can find strength in each other's stories.

Kindness, like a radiant beam of light, has the power to penetrate even the darkest of times. Throughout my journey, I was touched by countless acts of kindness – from small gestures like a friendly smile or a handwritten card to grand acts of generosity like fundraisers and community support. These acts reminded me that even in the face of adversity, the human spirit can rise above through compassion and empathy.

The legacy I hope to leave behind is one of courage and resilience, infused with a touch of kindness. It's about teaching future generations to find their inner strength, to embrace their vulnerabilities, and to inspire others through their own unique journeys. It's about demonstrating that even in the darkest moments, hope can be found in the smallest of actions and the unwavering belief in the power of the human spirit.

I often think about the young children I meet, their faces filled with a mixture of fear and curiosity as they embark on their own cancer journeys. I see in their eyes the same spark of resilience I discovered within myself. I want to empower them to find their own inner strength, to believe in their ability to heal, and to know that they are not alone.

This is the legacy I am building – a legacy of hope, courage, and resilience. It's a legacy that transcends personal experiences and reaches out to touch the lives of others, leaving behind a trail of inspiration and strength that will continue to shine long after I'm gone.

As I look back on my journey, I realize that the greatest gift I received wasn't just my own healing, but the opportunity to become a beacon of hope for others. My story, like a flickering candle, is meant to illuminate the path for those who need guidance, to remind them that even in the darkest of times, there is always light to be found.

The legacy of courage and resilience is not something we inherit; it's something we build, brick by brick, day by day. It's about the choices we make, the actions we take, and the impact we have on the world around us. It's about leaving behind a legacy of hope that will continue to shine long after we're gone. And that, my friends, is a legacy worth striving for.

I am not just a cancer survivor; I am a storyteller, a beacon of hope, and a torchbearer for future generations. My journey is a testament to the power of the human spirit, the strength of community, and the boundless potential for resilience. It is my hope that by sharing my story, I can inspire others to embrace their own journeys with courage, determination, and unwavering hope.

The legacy of courage and resilience is not about simply surviving; it's about thriving, about finding beauty in the midst of challenges, and about using our experiences to make a positive impact on the world. It's about recognizing that we all have the power to create a better future, a future filled with hope, compassion, and the unwavering belief in the human spirit's ability to overcome any obstacle.

Every time I share my story, I plant a seed of hope. My hope is that these seeds will take root, grow into strong and resilient trees, and spread their branches of inspiration far and wide, creating a world where courage and resilience are not just aspirations, but realities for all.

I believe that each of us has the potential to leave a legacy of courage and resilience. It may not be through grand gestures or sweeping statements, but through the simple act of being present, of offering a kind word, of showing empathy and understanding. It's about embracing the power of human connection and using our own experiences to uplift and inspire others.

The journey of overcoming cancer was a transformative experience that reshaped my perspective on life. It taught me to appreciate the simple joys, to cherish the moments with loved ones, and to find strength in my vulnerability. I discovered that healing is not just a physical process, but a journey of the soul, a rediscovery of self, and a reawakening of hope.

The legacy I hope to leave behind is not a monument to my own struggle, but a testament to the power of the human spirit, the strength of community, and the unwavering belief in the capacity for resilience. It's a legacy that transcends personal experiences and reaches out to touch the lives of others, leaving behind a trail of inspiration and strength that will continue to shine long after I'm gone.

The journey of overcoming cancer has been a profound one, but it has also been a deeply enriching one. It has opened my eyes to the beauty and fragility of life, the importance of human connection, and the boundless potential for healing and growth.

I believe that every individual has the power to leave a legacy of courage and resilience. It's a legacy that is built through our actions, our words, and the impact we have on the world around us. It's a legacy that inspires others to find their own strength, to embrace their vulnerabilities, and to believe in the power of hope.

I encourage you to embrace your own journey, to find your own inner strength, and to share your light with the world. Together, we can create a world where courage and resilience are not just aspirations, but realities for all.

A MESSAGE OF HOPE
FOR THE FUTURE

The journey through cancer, while challenging, is not about reaching the finish line and forgetting everything that happened. It's about embracing the lessons learned, carrying the strength gained, and sharing the light of hope that shines brighter than ever. It's about realizing that while the battle may be over, the fight for a brighter future continues.

Just like the sun rises each morning, casting its golden rays over a new day, our lives can be filled with a renewed sense of purpose and direction. We may have faced storms, endured darkness, and felt the weight of fear, but we emerged stronger, more resilient, and with a deeper understanding of life's preciousness.

The future is a canvas waiting to be painted with vibrant colors of hope, dreams, and possibilities. It's a chance to rewrite our story, not as survivors of cancer, but as individuals who have overcome adversity and emerged as beacons of strength and inspiration.

Each day offers a fresh start, a new opportunity to embrace life with gratitude and enthusiasm. We can choose to see the world with fresh eyes, marveling at the simplest joys, and appreciating the beauty that surrounds us. Every sunrise is a reminder that we are alive, that we have a chance to make a difference, to share our story, and to empower others.

Our journey through cancer has given us a unique perspective, a deeper understanding of the human spirit's capacity for resilience, and the importance of connecting with others. We can use this newfound knowledge to create a ripple effect of hope, spreading kindness, compassion, and support to those who need it most.

We can become mentors, guides, and champions for those still facing their own battles. We can share our stories, offering encouragement, strength, and a sense of solidarity. We can join hands with others, creating a community of hope and resilience, where no one feels alone.

The future holds countless opportunities to make a difference. We can pursue our passions, embrace new adventures, and contribute to the world in ways that inspire others. We can create a legacy of courage, strength, and hope, leaving behind a trail of light that illuminates the path for those who come after us.

It's not about forgetting the past, but about embracing the present and shaping a brighter future. It's about choosing to live with purpose, with intention, and with a heart filled with hope and gratitude.

Imagine a world where every survivor of cancer is seen not as a victim, but as a victor, a source of strength, and an inspiration to others. Imagine a world where the scars of our battles become badges of honor, reminders of our resilience, and symbols of our triumph over adversity.

This is the future we can create, not just for ourselves, but for generations to come. It's a future where the light of hope shines brighter than ever, guiding us all towards a world filled with healing, compassion, and a deep appreciation for the precious gift of life.

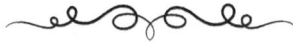

APPENDIX

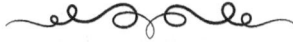

resources for young cancer patients and their families:

National Cancer Institute: Provides information and support for cancer patients and their families.
St. Jude Children's Research Hospital: Dedicated to finding cures and saving children with cancer.
Make-A-Wish Foundation: Grants wishes to children with critical illnesse.

This book is a testament to the power of love, support, and resilience, and I am deeply grateful to the countless individuals who have played a vital role in my journey.

This book is a blend of fact and fiction. A book that heavily leans towards factual information, drawing from real events and people, but was utilized some creative storytelling techniques to enhance the narrative, without including outright fictional elements that would classify it as a "fiction" which blends fact and fiction; essentially.

First and foremost, I would like to express my heartfelt thanks to my family and friends. Your unwavering love, strength, and understanding have been my anchor throughout this challenging experience.

I am eternally grateful to the exceptional medical professionals who provided me with exceptional care and compassion. Your skill, dedication, and unwavering belief in my recovery have been instrumental in my healing.

I also want to acknowledge the incredible strength and resilience of the other young cancer patients and survivors I have met along the way. Your stories of courage and hope inspire me every day.

To the organizations dedicated to supporting children with cancer and their families, thank you for your tireless work. Your efforts make a real difference in the lives of so many.

Finally, I want to thank my readers for taking the time to embark on this journey with me. I hope this book offers you strength, hope, and a reminder that even in the face of adversity, the human spirit can find its way to light.